Experimental and Clinical Immunogenetics

KARGER

Printed in Switzerland on acid-free paper by Reinhardt Druck, Basel

Appears quarterly: 1 volume per year (4 issues)

Guidelines for Authors

Experimental and
Clinical
Immunogenetics

Editorial policy

The journal publishes original research reports (generally limited to 8 printed pages), short communications (generally limited to 3 printed pages), and review articles. Appropriately brief manuscripts, intended for rapid publication, must be marked 'short communication'. Research reports require subdivisions of abstract, introduction, materials and methods, results, and discussion; short communications need not have subtitles. Authors interested in preparing a review article should first query the Editor (K. Bauer).

Submission

Only original papers written in English are considered and should be sent to:

Editor-in-Chief
PD Dr. K. Bauer
Postfach 101.560
D-69005 Heidelberg (Germany)

Representative for Japan
Prof. Dr. Hisao Takizawa, MD
Department of Legal Medicine
Toyama Medical and Pharmaceutical University
2630 Sugitani
Toyama-shi 930-01 (Japan)

Representative for North America
Prof. Dr. J.J. Marchalonis
Department of Microbiology and Immunology
Health Sciences Center
University of Arizona
Tucson, AZ 85724 (USA)

Representative for Scandinavia
Niels Ødum, MD, DSci.
Associate Professor
Institute of Medical Microbiology and Immunology
University of Copenhagen
Blegdamsvej 3c
DK-2200 Copenhagen N (Denmark)

Manuscripts should be submitted in quadruplicate (with four sets of illustrations of which one is an original), typewritten double-spaced on one side of the paper, with a wide margin.

Conditions

All manuscripts are subject to editorial review. Manuscripts are received with the explicit understanding that they are not under simultaneous consideration by any other publication. Submission of an article for publication implies the transfer of the copyright from the author to the publisher upon acceptance. Accepted papers become the permanent property of 'Experimental and Clinical Immunogenetics' and may not be reproduced by any means, in whole or in part, without the written consent of the publisher. It is the author's responsibility to obtain permission to reproduce illustrations, tables, etc. from other publications.

Arrangement

Title page: The first page of each paper should indicate the title (main title underlined), the authors' names, and the institute where the work was conducted. A short title for use as running head as well as the full address of the author to whom correspondence should be sent are also required.

Full address: The exact postal address complete with postal code must be given at the bottom of the title page. Please also supply phone and fax numbers, as well as your e-mail address.

Key words: For indexing purposes, a list of 3–10 key words in English is essential.

Abstract: Each paper needs an abstract of up to 10 lines.

Small type: Paragraphs which can or must be set in smaller type (case histories, test methods, etc.) should be indicated with a 'p' (petit) in the margin on the left-hand side.

Footnotes: Avoid footnotes. When essential, they are numbered consecutively and typed at the foot of the appropriate page.

Tables and illustrations: Tables and illustrations (both numbered in Arabic numerals) should be prepared on separate sheets. Tables require a heading and figures a legend, also prepared on a separate sheet. For the reproduction of illustrations, only good drawings and original photographs can be accepted; negatives or photocopies cannot be used. Due to technical reasons, figures with a screen background should not be submitted. When possible, group several illustrations on one block for reproduction (max. size 144 × 196 mm) or provide crop marks. On the back of each illustration, indicate its number, the author's name, and 'top' with a soft pencil.

Color illustrations: Up to 6 color illustrations per page can be integrated with the text at the reduced price of CHF 660.– / USD 545.00 per page. Color illustrations are reproduced at the author's expense.

References: In the text identify references by Arabic numerals [in square brackets]. Material submitted for publication but not yet accepted should be noted as 'unpublished data' and not be included in the reference list. The list of references should include only those publications which are cited in the text. Do not alphabetize; number references in the order in which they are first mentioned in the text. The surnames of the authors followed by initials should be given. There should be no punctuation other than a comma to separate the authors. Cite all authors, 'et al.' is not sufficient. Abbreviate journal names according to the Index Medicus system. (Also see International Committee of Medical Journal Editors: Uniform requirements for manuscripts submitted to biomedical journals. Br Med J 1988;296:401–405.)

Examples

(a) Papers published in periodicals: Sun J, Koto H, Chung KF: Interaction of ozone and allergen challenges on bronchial responsiveness and inflammation in sensitised guinea pigs. Int Arch Allergy Immunol 1997; 112: 191–195.

(b) Monographs: Matthews DE, Farewell VT: Using and Understanding Medical Statistics, ed 3, revised. Basel, Karger, 1996.

(c) Edited books: Parren PWHI, Burton DR: Antibodies against HIV-1 from phage display libraries: Mapping of an immune response and progress towards antiviral immunotherapy; in Capra JD (ed): Antibody Engineering. Chem Immunol. Basel, Karger, 1997, vol 65, pp 18–56.

Page charges

There is no page charge for papers of 7 or fewer printed pages (including tables, illustrations and references). Each additional complete or partial page is charged to the author at CHF 275.– / USD 196.00. The allotted size of a paper is equal to approx. 15 manuscript pages (including tables, illustrations and references).

Galley proofs

Unless indicated otherwise, galley proofs are sent to the first-named author and should be returned with the least possible delay. Alterations made in galley proofs, other than the correction of printer's errors, are charged to the author. No page proofs are supplied.

Reprints

Order forms and a price list are sent with the galley proofs. Orders submitted after the issue is printed are subject to considerably higher prices.

KARGER

Fax + 41 61 306 12 34
E-Mail karger@karger.ch
www.karger.com

The Guidelines for Authors are available at:
www.karger.com/journals/eci/eci_gl.htm

Experimental and Clinical
Immunogenetics

General Information

Publication data: 'Experimental and Clinical Immunogenetics' is published 4 times annually. Volume 15 with 4 issues appears in 1998.

Subscription rates: Subscriptions run for a full calendar year. Prices are given per volume.
Personal subscription:
Subscription + postage and handling
CHF 193.– + CHF 15.70 Europe
CHF 193.– + CHF 23.70 Overseas
USD 147.50 + USD 15.70
(Must be in the name of, billed to, and paid by an individual. Order must be marked 'personal subscription'.)
Institutional subscription:
Subscription + postage and handling
CHF 386.– + CHF 19.60 Europe
CHF 386.– + CHF 29.60 Overseas
USD 295.00 + USD 19.60
Airmail postage: CHF 24.–, USD 20.00.
(Extra per volume.)
Discount subscription prices:
EFI; Japanese Soc. for Immunology; Ges. für Immunologie.

Advertising: Correspondence and rate requests should be addressed to the Publisher.

Change of address: Both old and new address should be sent to the subscription source.

Microforms: Please direct all enquiries and orders to: University Microfilms Inc.
300 North Zeeb Road, P.O. Box 1346
Ann Arbor, MI 48106-1346 (USA)

Subscription orders: Orders can be placed at agencies, bookstores, directly with the
Publisher S. Karger AG, P.O. Box
CH–4009 Basel (Switzerland)
or with any of the following distributors:
Deutschland: S. Karger GmbH, Postfach
D–79095 Freiburg
France: Librairie Luginbühl
36, bd de Latour-Maubourg
F–75007 Paris
Great Britain, Ireland: S. Karger Publishers
58 Grove Hill Road
Tunbridge Wells, Kent TN1 1SP
USA: S. Karger Publishers, Inc.
26 West Avon Road, P.O. Box 529
Farmington, CT 06085
India, Bangladesh, Sri Lanka:
S. Karger India Subscription Agency
B–5/132 Safdarjung Enclave
New Delhi 110029
Japan: Katakura Libri, Inc.
Take 1 Bldg, 2nd Floor
4-5-7 Yushima, Bunkyo-ku
Tokyo 113

Single issues and back volumes: Information can be obtained through the Publisher.

Book Reviews: Books are accepted for review by special agreement.

Bibliographic indices: This journal is regularly listed in bibliographic services, including *Current Contents®*.

Copying: This journal has been registered with the Copyright Clearance Center (CCC), as indicated by the code appearing on the first page of each article.
For readers in the US, this code signals consent for copying of articles for personal or internal use, or for the personal or internal use of specific clients, provided that the stated fee is paid per copy directly to
Copyright Clearance Center Inc.
222 Rosewood Drive
Danvers, MA 01923 (USA).
A copy of the first page of the article must accompany payment. Consent does not extend to copying for general distribution, for promotion, for creating new works, or for resale. In these cases, specific written permission must be obtained from the copyright owner,
S. Karger AG, P.O. Box
CH–4009 Basel (Switzerland).

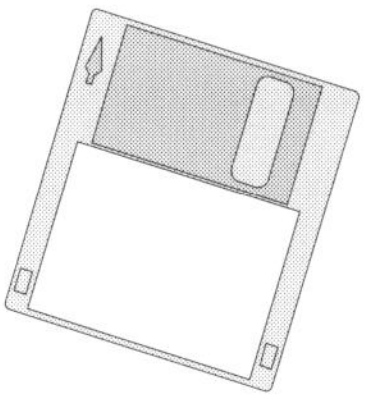

Disk Submission

A **comprehensive version** of these guidelines for the **submission of manuscripts and illustrations on disk** can be accessed online under **www.karger.com/journals/disksub.htm** or requested as a leaflet from the editorial department.

Please follow the general rules on style and arrangement in the **"Guidelines for Authors"** of the journal. Submit a **double-spaced printout** of your manuscript matching the file on disk exactly.

Technical Information

Store only data pertinent to this manuscript. Include your fonts (screen and printer fonts for Macintosh).
For a **text only** manuscript, use a 3.5 inch disk. For **text and illustrations,** use 3.5 or 5.25 Magneto Optical Disc; CD-ROM (DOS or hybrid); iomage Zip/DOS (100 MB), or 44 MB, 88 MB or 200 MB SyQuest. Compress extensive data using ZIP format.

Data Description

Label your disk with the **title of the journal or book** for which it is submitted; a **short version** of the paper's title; your **name,** postal and e-mail address, fax and phone number; **hard and software** used, including the version; and the **complete list of the file names.** File names consist of eight characters before the dot identifying the file and three characters after the dot identifying the application.

Text and Format

The **preferred word-processing package is MS-Word.** Other commonly used PC text programs and ASCII formats are accepted.
Update your data when you revise subsequent to the reviewer's or editor's decision and mark revisions clearly. Manuscripts accepted for publication are subject to **copy editing:** changes and/or questions will be marked in the manuscript, which will be returned to you with your disk and the galley proofs for checking.
Enter your text continuously flush left. Do not use any layout functions. Do not split words at the end of a line. **Do not use indentations.** Use a blank line before and a hard return at the end of paragraphs. **Arrange headings flush left.** Insert only **one space after punctuation marks.** Insert Greek letters, mathematical symbols etc. with your word-processing program. Use **boldface and italics** as well as sub- and superscript where appropriate. **Tables are part of the text** and should be placed at the end of the text file. Separate the individual parts of a table by lines. Use the tabulator instead of spaces. Format operation data on one line in the same column. **Legends to illustrations are part of the text** and should also be listed at the end of the text file.

Illustrations

Store illustrations as separate files: do not embed them in your text. Export **line drawings/vector graphics** as TIF, EPS or WMF format. Use Photoshop for processing and retouching **scanned half-tone images.** Save the original scan and the processed version. Export **black and white or color images** as TIF or EPS format in their anticipated size in print.
For detailed information on how to submit illustration data on disk please consult the leaflet or **www.karger.com/journals/disksub.htm.**

KARGER

KI 98 DISK

Fax + 41 61 306 12 34
E-Mail karger@karger.ch
www.karger.com

The Journal Home Page is available at:
www.karger.com/journals/eci

Experimental and Clinical Immunogenetics

VIIth Complement Genetics Workshop and Conference

Mainz, May 21–23, 1998

Proceedings

Editors
Peter M. Schneider, Mainz
Christian Rittner, Mainz
Gottfried Mauff, Hamburg
Reinhard Würzner, Innsbruck

21 figures, 21 tables, 1999

KARGER
Basel · Freiburg · Paris · London · New York · New Delhi · Bangkok · Singapore · Tokyo · Sydney

KARGER

S. Karger
Medical and Scientific Publishers
Basel · Freiburg · Paris · London
New York · New Delhi · Bangkok
Singapore · Tokyo · Sydney

Drug Dosage
The authors and the publisher have exerted every effort to ensure that drug selection and dosage set forth in this text are in accord with current recommendations and practice at the time of publication. However, in view of ongoing research, changes in government regulations, and the constant flow of information relating to drug therapy and drug reactions, the reader is urged to check the package insert for each drug for any change in indications and dosage and for added warnings and precautions. This is particularly important when the recommended agent is a new and/or infrequently employed drug.

Printed in Switzerland on acid-free paper by
Reinhardt Druck, Basel
ISBN 3–8055–6813–4

Experimental and Clinical Immunogenetics

Contents Vol. 15, No. 4, 1998

KARGER

Fax+41 61 306 12 34
E-Mail karger@karger.ch
www.karger.com

Access to full text and tables of contents, including tentative ones for forthcoming issues:
www.karger.com/journals/eci/eci_bk.htm

Editorial

Experimental and Clinical Immunogenetics

Exp Clin Immunogenet 1998;15:201–202

Peter M. Schneider[a]
Christian Rittner[a]
Gottfried Mauff[b]
Reinhard Würzner[c]

[a] Institute of Legal Medicine, Johannes Gutenberg University, Mainz,
[b] State Institute of Hygiene, Hamburg, Germany, and
[c] Institute of Hygiene, Leopold Franzens University, Innsbruck, Austria

VIIth Complement Genetics Workshop and Conference

Proceedings
Mainz, May 21–23, 1998

It is often difficult to identify the beginning of a scientific field. In this issue, Chester Alper, who has personally made many key contributions to its advancement, has reviewed the dawn of complement genetics, revealing that already 80 years ago, a complement-deficient guinea pig was identified, and has also recalled that it was only 30 years ago when the first description of a genetic polymorphism was discovered independently by three groups for the third component and published in the United States in 1968 and a year later in the former East Germany. These observations have initiated a new field of genetic research. The first international workshop on complement genetics was held in Bonn, Germany, in 1972. It focussed on a single component, C3. Twenty scientists discussed methods, nomenclature, formal and population genetics of C3 polymorphism. Thereafter, complement genetics workshops have been held in Cambridge in 1977, in Cologne in 1979, in Boston in 1982 and in 1986, and in Mainz in 1989 and very recently, in 1998, again on the banks of the Rhine, only 150 km away from Bonn, the cradle of this workshop series.

The results of the reference typings of the recent 1998 workshop have been compiled in this issue. Many reference typing laboratories all around the world took part in comparative investigations on selected complement components. It was the aim of this workshop, as of the previous ones, to update most of the known complement polymorphisms by standardising reference typing and proposing nomenclature revisions. Emphasis has been laid on complement components of the major histocompatibility complex (MHC) class III cluster, especially C4, as before, on components of the terminal complement complex (TCC or MAC) gene cluster (C6, C7 and C9), and on complement receptor 1 (CR1) of the regulators of complement activation (RCA) gene cluster. For C2, C8, factor I, and other components of the RCA cluster, we have to refer to the previous proceedings [1].

High voltage agarose gel electrophoresis and isoelectric focusing, combined with hae-

KARGER

Fax + 41 61 306 12 34
E-Mail karger@karger.ch
www.karger.com

0254–9670/98/0154–0201$17.50/0

Accessible online at:
http://BioMedNet.com/karger

Reinhard Würzner, MD, PhD
Institute of Hygiene
Fritz-Pregl-Strasse 3, A–6020 Innsbruck (Austria)
Tel. +43 512 507 3426, Fax +43 512 507 2870
E-Mail Reinhard.Wuerzner@uibk.ac.at

molytic overlay, immunoblotting, or immunofixation have, for years, been the most important technique for the assessment of complement allotypes. Despite the fact that allospecific monoclonal antibodies are available for C4, C3 and C7, genetic typing of polymorphic variants by electrophoretic methods has maintained its dominant position. However, using recombinant DNA technology, tremendous progress has been accomplished over the last 15 years in the definition of the genetic basis of the complement system, including polymorphisms and deficiencies. Most of the approximately 40 genes coding for C components or subunits, receptors and regulators have been cloned, sequenced and assigned to chromosomal locations. Protocols for both protein and DNA typing methods have recently been compiled and discussed in great detail – despite some overlap, both publications 'complement' each other quite well [2, 3].

Apart from the historical overview and the reference typing reports, this issue also contains reviews of selected presentations at the meeting covering

- gene organisation and evolution of the MHC class III complement genes (Yu),
- deficiency of C1q and its implications for development of autoimmune disease (Botto),
- gene organisation and evolution of the terminal complement genes (Hobart),
- deficiencies of terminal complement genes (Fukumori).

An overview of these and other aspects of the meeting, including the application of polymorphisms to a wide range of problems, such as association with disease, structure-function relationships, as well as phylogenetic and population genetic studies, is concurrently published elsewhere [4].

We hope that this issue will help the workshop participants review the meeting and assist the interested reader in obtaining the latest information on complement genetics. Scientists working with a particular component may contact the authors for any questions, particularly on polymorphisms and deficiencies both on the protein and on the molecular level. We especially hope to encourage young scientists to join us in this exciting task and conclude with the optimistic view that it will not take another nine years before we have a chance to meet again at the VIIIth Complement Genetics Workshop.

Last but not least we would like to acknowledge gratefully the financial support we have received for organising this meeting. The VIIth Complement Genetics Workshop was sponsored the Deutsche Forschungsgemeinschaft (DFG), the Academy of Sciences and Literature in Mainz, as well as by travel grants from the BIOMED 2 concerted action (Complement in Infection and Chronic Disease, secretary M.R. Daha, Leiden) via the European Complement Network (ECN, secretary R. Würzner, Innsbruck).

The Editors

References

1 Rittner C, Hauptmann G, Mauff G, Schneider PM (eds): Proceedings of the VIth complement genetics workshop and conference. Complement Inflamm 1990;7:173–314.

2 Schneider PM, Rittner C: Complement genetics; in Dodds AW, Sim RB (eds): Complement – A Practical Approach. Oxford, Oxford University Press, 1997, pp 165–198.

3 Mauff G, Würzner R: Complement genetics; in Herzenberg LA, Weir DM, Herzenberg LA, Blackwell C (eds): Weir's Handbook of Experimental Immunology. Oxford, Blackwell, 1996, vol 2, pp 77.1–77.11.

4 Schneider PM, Würzner R: Complement genetics: Biological implications of polymorphisms and deficiencies. Immunol Today 1999;20: 2–5.

Experimental and Clinical Immunogenetics

Exp Clin Immunogenet 1998;15:203–212

Received: July 15, 1998
Accepted: September 14, 1998

Chester A. Alper

The Center for Blood Research
and the Department of Pediatrics,
Harvard Medical School,
Boston, Mass., USA

A History of Complement Genetics

Key Words
Complement
Genetic polymorphisms
Inherited deficiencies
History

Abstract
After a brief review of the history of the complement system from the original observations in the 1880s, the history of complement genetics is outlined, beginning in 1919 with the recognition of the complement-deficient guinea pig. A highly personal view is then presented of the early days of the discovery of human complement structural gene polymorphisms and deficiencies, particularly those of C3, BF and factor I. Finally, some recent work based on features in the DNA of the MHC-encoded complement genes is outlined that sheds some light on their evolution.

It is not my intention to review exhaustively the history of complement genetics. Rather, I will try to describe my personal view and experiences in the early days that preceded and immediately followed the first complement genetics meeting in Bonn. To complete this picture, I will try to trace the origins of complement research in general and complement genetics in particular and end with a recent study from my laboratory that relates to some of our early work.

It is often difficult to identify the beginning of a scientific field. For example, when did our knowledge of the complement system begin? Was it when John Hunter [1] observed that blood from both old and young subjects left at the room temperature of an English summer took a long time to become putrid? If we reframe the question to include the requirement that the beginning have some temporal continuity with later work, then perhaps we can regard its having occurred in the report by Grohmann [2] in 1884 that cell-free blood plasma was capable of killing bacteria and other microorganisms. Perhaps equally seminal was the observation by Nuttall, an American working in Göttingen and Breslau [3], that treatment with fresh plasma produced morphologic changes in target microorganisms and that bactericidal activity was

KARGER
Fax + 41 61 306 12 34
E-Mail karger@karger.ch
www.karger.com

Accessible online at:
http://BioMedNet.com/karger

Chester A. Alper
The Center for Blood Research and the Department of Pediatrics
Harvard Medical School, Boston, MA 02115 (USA)
Tel. +1 617 278 3333, Fax +1 617 278 3493
E-Mail alper@cbr.med.harvard.edu

abolished by heating the plasma at 55 °C for 1 h. The exuberance of the brilliant early deciphering of the complement system that took place, largely in Germany and France, over the next 30 years, laid the groundwork for all later investigation and almost discovered the alternative pathway in 1913 [4], only to die down almost completely after World War I. A little over 30 years after the beginning of complement research, in 1919 in the United States at the Vermont Agricultural Experiment Station in Burlington, the first observations in complement genetics were made by Moore [5] and Hyde [6] in the description of the complement-deficient guinea pig. Most remarkably, this deficiency was the first instance of an inherited defect of any protein in a mammal. After a number of elegant experiments, the stain of guinea pigs was lost before the renaissance of complement research after World War II in America and Europe, so that we shall likely never know which complement protein was, in fact, missing in these animals. We do know that the defect was inherited as an autosomal recessive trait with detectable expression in the heterozygote and that the complement component in question did not cross the placenta in either direction [6].

Inbred and wild mice defective in hemolytic complement were noted by Tachibana et al. [7]. Independently, an inherited absence of a serum protein, MuB1, was reported by Cinader and Dubiski [8]. Two was put together with two [9] and it was clear that the two defects reflected homozygous deficiency of C5, which affects about half the strains of inbred mice. Rabbits homozygous for deficiency in C6 [10] turned out to be fairly common (around 5% of rabbits offered for sale in the market at Xochimilco in Mexico City) [11].

The next milestone was in human complement genetics with the recognition by Donaldson and Evans [12] and Kagen and Becker [13] in 1963 that patients with hereditary angioedema had an autosomal dominant defect in the inhibitor of the esterase of the first component of complement. A few years later, Klemperer et al. [14] demonstrated clearly that the deficiency of C2 noted in an immunologist who tried to use his own serum as a source of normal complement [15] was inherited as an autosomal recessive trait. Some C2-deficient persons had systemic-lupus-erythematosus-like disease [16] and this has also proved to be true of persons deficient in other classical pathway components.

Complement genetics up to this point was concerned with a few rare deficiency states in animals and humans. These were of great help in aiding our understanding of the part played by complement in the clearance of immune complexes. But the great potential for a role of complement proteins and genes in population genetics or forensics was completely unrealized.

As with so many scientific fields, technical advances were the engines of progress. The introduction of new electrophoretic techniques using starch, agar, agarose and polyacrylamide gels and isoelectrofocusing in polyacrylamide gel facilitated the recognition of human protein genetic diversity. By the late 1960s, through the work of Harry Harris in London, Oliver Smithies in Toronto, Ontario and Madison, Wisconsin, Rune Grubb and Anna-Brita Laurell, Carl-Bertil Laurell and Magne Fagerhol and Jan Hirschfeld in Sweden and many others, common polymorphisms were recognized in a score or so of human blood proteins [17]. The time was ripe for the application of these techniques to proteins of the complement system. Since C3 is the most abundant of the complement proteins and easily visible in directly stained electrophoretic patterns of fresh serum, it is not surprising that rare variants of these were the first to be detected by us in agarose gel [18] and Wieme and Demeulenaere [19] in agar gel. I had obtained a handmade agarose gel electrophoresis apparatus from Carl-Bertil Laurell, who was my mentor during an NIH postdoctoral fellowship with him and Jan Waldenström in Malmö, Sweden, in the early 1960s. The common polymorphism in C3 was discovered independently by Richard Propp and me [20], by Edwin Azen and Oliver Smithies [21], who were applying a newly-devised high-voltage starch gel electrophoresis system and noticed a set of polymorphic bands in fresh but not aged serum, and by Rose and Geserick [22] in the former East Berlin, who had to produce the hydrolyzed starch for their experiments themselves. They noted the post-transferrin polymorphism in aged or complement-activated serum that was, in fact, manifest in the major breakdown product of C3 in serum, C3c. As a footnote to the history of the Cold War, Western journals were very slow in arriving (if they arrived at all) behind the Iron Curtain so that when Rose and Geserick reported their finding, neither the previous year's *Journal of Clinical Investigation* nor *Science* had arrived in East Berlin. It was Christian Rittner, who had emigrated from East to West Germany some years earlier and was an old friend of Günther Geserick's, who alerted him to the other publications. In another accident of history, while our first paper on C3 polymorphism was still in press, I presented our preliminary findings on the first patient, TJ, with factor I deficiency at a meeting of the American Society of Hematology in New York. Edwin Azen was in the audience and, after the presentation, eagerly offered to type the C3 of this patient (whose C3 was being converted and consumed by spontaneous activation of the alternative complement pathway). I felt very sorry to have to tell him we already knew the patient's C3 type.

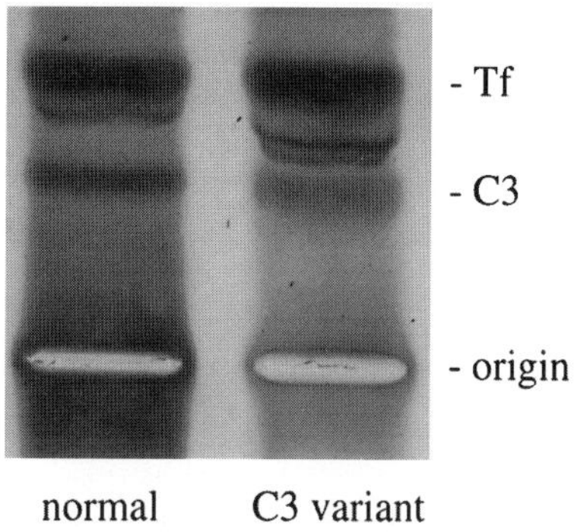

Fig. 1. Agarose gel electrophoresis on a Laurell apparatus in Ca^{2+}-containing barbital buffer at pH 8.6 of fresh standard (normal) serum (left) and C3 F1-containing (C3 variant) serum (right). The right-hand blurred pattern led us to the study of C3 genetics.

The route by which we came to recognize the common polymorphism in C3 was indirect. Using Laurell's agarose gel electrophoretic apparatus, the C3 band in the first serum sample that we recognized as having a rare C3 variant was merely wider and more blurred than other samples sent in for clinical serum protein analysis (fig. 1). It was clear that we had to run the samples longer in order to resolve what was going on. When we examined samples from this patient and her family members in prolonged agarose gel electrophoresis on the original apparatus, it became evident that variant patterns came in two varieties, wide and narrow (fig. 2). It is inconceivable to me now that we could not understand the meaning of this for some weeks. I vividly remember the moment of insight. As has often happened to me since, it occurred at a concert. It could also have happened, and subsequently has, for other scientific puzzles, while looking at art. Once realizing that the wide and narrow patterns reflected the com-

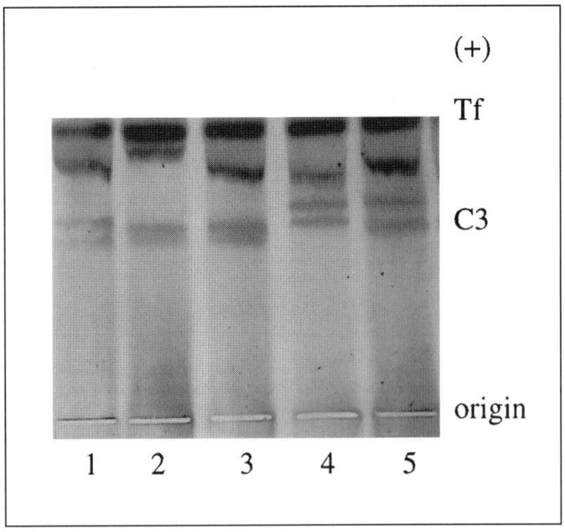

Fig. 2. A longer separation on a Laurell apparatus of sera containing (from left to right) (1) C3 FS1 (wide), (2) SS1 (narrow), (3) SS1 (narrow), (4) F1F (narrow), and (5) F1S (wide) patterns.

mon polymorphism, it was easy to check the inherited putative fast and slow forms of C3. Seeing the differences in a sample with a single common gene product in relation to the internal standard of what was eventually called C3 F1 or S1 and being able to type the common form without this standard was a technical problem that we solved very simply by redesigning Laurell's agarose gel electrophoresis apparatus to run samples the long way. This permitted even longer runs and the sought-after complete definition of the common slow and fast C3 variants [20].

Our first application of the C3 polymorphism to a scientific problem was in the analysis of a young patient who was discovered by mistake to have a half-normal C3 serum level. He was admitted to the Children's Hospital in Boston for failure to thrive. Pursuing every lead and because the patient's father had a thyroid problem, the patient's serum was sent to the laboratory for a BEI (butanol-extractable iodide). This was misread as β1C (an obsolete term for C3). An alert house officer noticed the half-normal value, obtained a repeat sample from the patient, as well as from his mother and a sister who had come to the clinic with him for a follow-up visit, even though it was decided that he had thrived after all. By chance all three had half-normal β1C levels. He then told Fred Rosen, with whom I was working closely, about the patient. Fred brought the samples to me, thinking they might have the same defect as TJ, whom we had just begun to study. The C3 types in this family provided the first evidence for a C3 null gene, albeit in heterozygotes only [23]. We arrogantly thought that homozygosity for deficiency of C3 must be lethal. Some time later, Arthur Rabson, then in Johannesburg, South Africa, now in Boston, wrote to me and to Fred Rosen, saying he had a patient with no detectable serum C3. I never answered a letter so fast in my life. Fred and I went to Johannesburg to work with Arthur on the first homozygous C3-deficient patient [24]. The C3 types in some cases were of the same pattern as we had found earlier in the heterozygote-only family, confirming the presence of a silent C3 gene. In the greater scheme of things, it was the fact that this patient and the homozygous factor-I-deficient patient TJ [25] both had strikingly increased susceptibility to infection by pyogenic bacteria that convinced us and the world that complement was more than a laboratory curiosity and had real relevance to human health.

Having the common genetic polymorphism in C3 made it possible to explore some basic physiologic facts about C3. Being at the Blood Grouping Laboratory gave us access to paired maternal-cord serum samples because of screening for anti-Rh. The finding that mother and child could differ in C3 type without a detectable trace of the other's C3 [26] showed that C3 did not cross the placenta in either direction. Since we had earlier shown that recipients of transplanted livers with different haptoglobin genetic types changed their types after several days to that of the donor, it was simple to test whether this was so for C3. The results were clear and demonstrated that, since no recipient C3 was detectable from several days after engraftment, the great bulk of C3 was made by hepatocytes [27]. Since that time, much evidence has been obtained that C3 can also be made by other cell types so that one must keep in mind that local synthesis may be of great importance.

As with almost all of our new findings, particularly in those days, the detection of the genetic polymorphism in factor B owed as much to chance as it did to any planning or cleverness on our part. Tom Boenisch, then of our lab, had been trained in Austria as a wine chemist but had been drawn to clinical chemistry and developed a passion for plasma proteins. He had isolated a protein from pooled and aged serum and characterized it with respect to molecular weight, amino acid composition and carbohydrate composition. Since it was particularly rich in glycine, he called it glycine-rich γ-glycoprotein (or, familiarly and by necessity, GGG) [28]. We raised an antiserum to it and were surprised to find that the antiserum reacted with a beta rather than a gamma mobility protein in fresh serum. After a few false starts, including questions of differences in Ca^{2+} binding, it became evident that GGG was a fragment of a native serum protein, which we promptly isolated, characterized and dubbed glycine-rich β-glycoprotein or GBG [29]. We soon found that both GGG and GBG reacted with antiserum to β_2-glycoprotein II, a protein described by Haupt and Heide of the Behringwerke a few years earlier [30]. Two further obervations soon helped to unravel the function of GBG. In fresh serum, GBG proved to be remarkably heat labile, cleaving into two fragments after brief incubation at 50°C, GGG and an α-mobility fragment we naturally called GAG. When I told Fred Rosen, who had worked as a medical student in Pillemer's lab in Cleveland, about this property, he immediately told me that I should learn something about the properdin pathway and ventured the opinion that GBG had the heat lability of the as yet unisolated factor B of that pathway [31]. We then observed that GBG instantaneously fragmented when incubated in TJ serum, leading us to postulate an enzyme, GBGase, for which the patient lacked an inhibitor [32]. Our work and that of Hans Müller-Eberhard and Otto Götze with C3 proactivator (C3PA), a protein necessary for the conversion of C3 by cobra venom factor [33], converged at the International Complement Workshop in Baltimore in 1971 where Irwin Lepow, formerly of the Pillemer group, publicly stated his conviction that GBG and C3PA were both factor B. Formal proof followed [34]. The relationship between the properdin (now the alternative) pathway of complement activation, factor B, C3 and the hereditary deficiency of factor I (C3b inactivator or conglutinogen activating factor or KAF) that was patient TJ's basic problem was finally sorted out in collaboration with Fred Rosen, Neil Abramson, Jim Jandl and Peter Lachmann [35–37].

By the time we had the antiserum that reacted with factor B, we could not resist the temptation to determine if it was genetically polymorphic. Fortunately, we now had prolonged agarose gel electrophoresis and we had earlier developed the technique of immunofixation [38] for the study of polymorphism in serum proteins. Our first antiserum was weak, so we had to use a second antibody to produce a usable pattern, but the rewards were immediate [39].

As an aside to the genetic polymorphism in GBG, now called BF, its fragmentation provided us with the opportunity to explore the molecular basis of its four common variants,

BF F, BF S, BF F1, and what we call BF S1, but others, noting that the distance between the main BF S to BF slow variant was about 70% of the BF S to BF F1 distance, call BF S0.7 [40]. The difference in viewpoint inherent in these two designations probably relates to the European desire for tidiness and an American lax practicality. The BF F/S polymorphism was detected in the Ba (GAG) fragment, whereas the BF F1/S1 polymorphism was in the Bb (GGG) fragment. Moreover, the Ba fragments of BF F1 and BF S1 carry the same Ba as BF S, suggesting that the mutations producing *BF*F1* and *BF*S1* occurred in a *BF*S* gene [39]. A major addition to the BF polymorphism was the recognition by two groups independently [41, 42] of the division by isoelectric focussing of *BF*F* into *BF*FA* and *BF*FB*. The BF FA/FB distinction was shown by Siemens et al. [43] to be in the Ba fragment. With the rapid development of DNA technology, including the facilitation of DNA sequencing, the molecular bases of the BF variant alleles have been worked out [44, 45] and, I am happy to say, our crude localizations have been proved correct.

Hal Allen, my predecessor at the Blood Grouping Lab and subsequently of the New York Blood Center, had been searching in vain for a decade for new linkages between human genetic markers. When I mentioned the 'new' BF polymorphism to him, he was immediately interested and we helped him set the system up. He hit pay dirt immediately with the BF-HLA linkage [46]. Around the same time, Henry Kunkel's group showed the linkage between C2 deficiency and HLA [47]. These two observations opened up a vast new area of scientific exploration. It was our finding the *BF*F1* marker in type 1 diabetes [48] that drew us inexorably into the MHC and determined the rest of my scientific career.

A major contribution, by Mike Hobart, in the early days of complement genetics was the introduction of functional overlay detection gels for complement proteins [49]. This technique and immunofixation greatly facilitated the study of complement genetics. Molecular DNA techniques came later and, of course, revolutionized the field.

Despite my current interests in MHC control of immune function of B cells, T cells, dendritic cells, NK cells and monocytes, I continue to be intrigued by complement genetics. In recent published work by Susan Simon, formerly of our lab, and Lennart Truedsson, a frequent working visitor in our lab, we have defined what we call complement RFLP constellations or CRC [50]. Because the four complement genes of the MHC occur in populations as conserved haplotypes or complotypes [47], variations in noncoding DNA should allow splitting of common complotypes such as SC31 (BF*S, C2*C, C4A*3, C4B*1) or SC30 (BF*S, C2*C, C4A*3, C4B*Q0). They should also provide some information on the evolution of the complotype region genes.

Based on 5 RFLP sites in the complement region [51–57] and the presence or absence of deletions (del) and duplications (dup) of C4 and CYP21 genes, it was possible to define 19 CRCs (of over 1000 theoretically possible) [50]. Remarkably, there are about 30 CRC-specified protein complotypes with frequencies of 0.01 or higher and 14 of 0.02 or higher in our Boston Caucasian population. Most important, we have clearly succeeded in 'splitting' the common complotypes. In attempting to dissect the evolution of the MHC complement genes, we reasoned that CRCs were most closely related evolutionarily if they shared the maximum number of DNA features. The direction of the relatedness was assigned on the basis of certain DNA or protein features being considered 'terminal'. For example, deletions or duplications were viewed as deriving from full haplotypes. C2*B

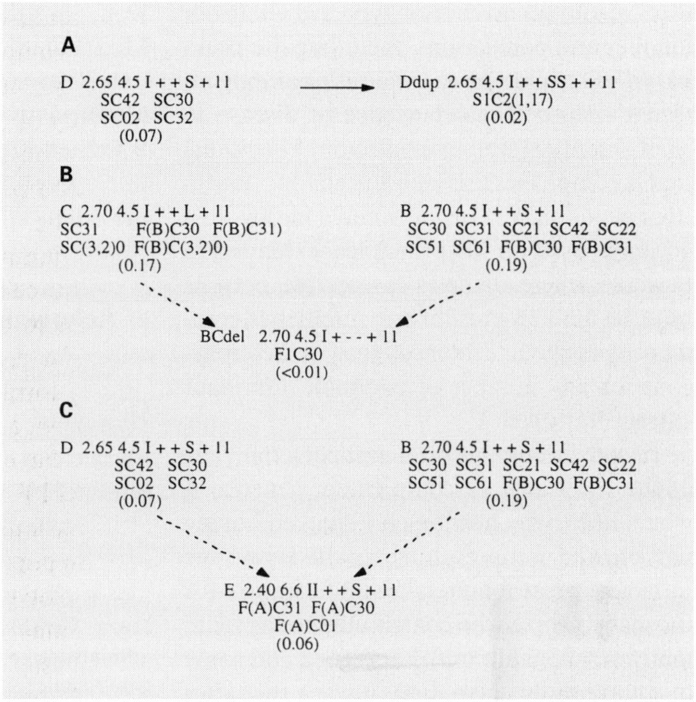

Fig. 3. Possible evolutionary relationships between complotype-RFLP constellations (CRC) in relation to generation of variation in BF alleles. The CRC are defined by an arbitrary letter, and the following RFLP (gene/restriction enzyme): *C2/Sst* I, *BF/Taq* I, 5′ *C4/Bgl* II, 5′ *C4/Taq* I, 3′ *C4 Xba* I/*Bam*H I. '+' indicates, in order, the presence and '–' the absence of *C4A, CYP21A, C4B* and *CYP21B*; '++' indicates a duplication of *C4B* or *CYP21B*. A short *C4B* gene is indicated by 'S' and a long one by 'L'. The approximate frequency of each CRC among normal Caucasian chromosomes is given in parentheses after the complotypes that are found in them. **A** CRC D, containing complotypes with *BF*S* and *BF*F(B)*, is postulated to have given rise to CRC Ddup with duplicated *C4B* and *CYP21B* and bearing a single complotype S1C2 (1,17) with *BF*S1*. **B** *BF*F1* in CRC BCdel could have arisen by deletion of *CYP21A* and *C4B* from either CRC B (with *BF*S* and *BF*F(B)*) or C (with only *BF*F(B)*). **C** The possible origin of *BF*FA* in CRC E from either *BF*S* in CRC D or CRC B or *BF*F(B)* in CRC B. CRC E differs from both CRC D and CRC B in three RFLP.

and C2*Q0 were deemed terminal derivations from C2*C. C4B*2 was considered to have arisen from C4B*1. Using these principles, figure 3 gives possible origins for *BF*S1*, *BF*F1*, *BF*FA* and *BF*FB*. The results are consistent with our earlier observations from electrophoretic analysis of fragments of factor B and the more recent sequence data.

I would like to close my highly selective and personal observations on the history of complement genetics with an affirmation of how my early experiences with genetic polymorphism in complement and other serum proteins have laid the foundation for very recent work that I and my colleagues have been doing with type 1 diabetes as a model of polygenic disease. Obviously, details about polygenic models are beyond the scope of this talk. What can be pointed out is that it is possible to predict all of the major puzzling features of the occurrence of type 1 diabetes in families and populations, including the peculiar MHC haplotype sharing ratios among affected siblings, the occurrence of disease in MHC-identical siblings and so on. The model that accomplishes this [submitted for publication] would make Gregor Mendel happy. It is entirely based on his principles, extended to the case where diabetes-susceptible persons must be homozygous for any number of common recessive and homozygous or heterozygous for any number of common dominant susceptibility genes.

In concluding this brief and personal view of the early days of complement genetics, I would like to say how much I enjoyed having participated in this exciting period. I continue to have a great fondness and admiration for the many people who contributed to the field, many of whom are in the audience and some of whom, sadly, have died. Among the latter are Irwin Lepow, Hans Müller-Eberhard, Manfred Mayer, Hal Allen, Rodney Porter, Don Shreffler, Henry Kunkel and Tommy Meo. I thank my good and old friends, Christian Rittner, Peter Schneider, and Gottfried Mauff, as well as my new friend, Reinhard Würzner, the organizers of this meeting, for this opportunity for me to bring back to life the events and people of those heady days.

Acknowledgments

The original observations reported here have been supported by NIH grant AI 14157 for the past 27 years. I gratefully acknowledge my many colleagues and collaborators, too numerous to list, who contributed so essentially to our work described here. I thank my technicians, and particularly my chief technicians, Diane Balavitch Banda, Debbie Marcus-Bagley, and the late Lillian Watson, without whom none of this would have been possible. Throughout the period described here, Louise Viehmann has provided superb secretarial and administrative support. Finally, I wish to thank my wife Natalie for unstinting support and for teaching me about art and thereby helping my science.

References

1 Hunter J: A Treatise on the Blood, Inflammation, and Gun-Shot Wounds. Philadelphia, Webster, 1817, pp 77–79.
2 Grohmann W: Über die Einwirkung des zellenfreien Blutplasma auf einige pflanzliche Microorganismen (schimmel-, spross-, pathogene und nichtpathogene Spaltpilze). Dorpat, C Mattiesen, 1884, p 34.
3 Nuttall G: Experimente über die bacterienfeindlichen Einflüsse des thierischen Körpers. Z Hyg 1888;4:353–394.
4 Browning CH, Mackie TJ: The relationship of the complementing action of fresh serum along with immune body to its haemolytic effect with cobra venom – a contribution on the structure of complement. Z Immun-Forsch 1913;17:1–20.
5 Moore HD: Complementary and opsonic functions in their relation to immunity. A study of the serum of guinea pigs naturally deficient in complement. J Immunol 1919;4:425–441.
6 Hyde RR: The complement deficient guinea pig: A study of an inheritable factor in immunity. Am J Hyg 1932;15:824–836.
7 Tachibana DK, Ulrich M, Rosenberg LT: The inheritance of hemolytic complement activity in CF-1 mice. J Immunol 1963;91:230–232.
8 Cinader B, Dubiski S: An alpha-globulin allotype in the mouse (MuB1). Nature 1963;200:781–782.
9 Nilsson UR, Müller-Eberhard HJ: Deficiency of the fifth component of complement in mice with an inherited complement defect. J Exp Med 1967;125:1–16.
10 Rother K, Rother U, Müller-Eberhard HJ, Nilsson UR: Deficiency of the sixth component of complement in rabbits with an inherited complement defect. J Exp Med 1966;124:773–785.
11 Biro CE, Ortega ML: Algunas características del sexto componente del complemento. Arch Inst Cardiol Mex 1966;36:166–168.
12 Donaldson VH, Evans RR: A biochemical abnormality in hereditary angioneurotic edema: Absence of serum inhibitor of C′1 esterase. Am J Med 1963;35:37–44.
13 Kagen LJ, Becker EL: Inhibition of permeability globulins by C1 esterase inhibitor (abstract). Fed Proc 1963;22:613.

14 Klemperer MR, Woodworth HC, Rosen FS, Austen KF: Hereditary deficiency of the second component of complement in man. J Clin Invest 1966;45:880–890.
15 Silverstein AM: Essential hypocomplementemia: Report of a case. Blood 1960;16:1338–1341.
16 Agnello V, de Bracco MME, Kunkel HG: Hereditary C2 deficiency with some manifestations of systemic lupus erythematosus. J Immunol 1972;108:837–840.
17 Giblett ER: Genetic Markers in Human Blood. Oxford, Blackwell, 1969.
18 Alper CA, Propp RP: An electrophoretic variant of human C′3 (abstract). Clin Res 1967;15:291.
19 Wieme RJ, Demeulenaere L: Genetically determined electrophoretic variant of the human complement component C′3. Nature 1967;214: 1042–1043.
20 Alper CA, Propp RP: Genetic polymorphism of the third component of human complement (C′3). J Clin Invest 1968;47:2181–2191.
21 Azen EA, Smithies O: Genetic polymorphism of C′3 (beta-1C-globulin) in human serum. Science 1968;162: 905–907.
22 Rose M, Geserick G: Ein neuer Serumproteinpolymorphismus. Pt. Erste Hinweise für eine genetische Steuerung. Acta Biol Med Germ 1969;23:351–356.
23 Alper CA, Propp RP, Klemperer MR, Rosen FS: Inherited deficiency of the third component of human complement (C′3). J Clin Invest 1969;48:553–557.
24 Alper CA, Colten HR, Rosen FS, Rabson AR, Macnab GM, Gear JSS: Homozygous deficiency of C3 in a patient with repeated infections. Lancet 1972;ii:1179–1181.
25 Alper CA, Abramson N, Johnston RB Jr, Jandl JH, Rosen FS: Increased susceptibility to infection associated with abnormalities of complement-mediated functions and of the third component of complement (C3). N Engl J Med 1970; 282:349–354.
26 Propp RP, Alper CA: C′3 synthesis in the human fetus and lack of transplacental passage. Science 1968;162: 672–673.
27 Alper CA, Johnson AM, Birtch AG, Moore FD: Human C′3: Evidence for the liver as the primary site of synthesis. Science 1969;163:286–288.
28 Boenisch T, Alper CA: Isolation and properties of a glycine-rich γ-glycoprotein of human serum. Biochim Biophys Acta 1970;214:135–140.
29 Boenisch T, Alper CA: Isolation and properties of a glycine-rich β-glycoprotein of human serum. Biochim Biophys Acta 1970;221:529–535.
30 Haupt H, Heide K: Isolierung und Eigenschaften eines Beta II-Glykoproteins aus Humanserum. Clin Chim Acta 1965;12:419–424.
31 Blum L, Pillemer L, Lepow IH: The properdin system and immunity. XIII. Assay and properties of heat labile serum factor (factor B) in the properdin system. Z Immunitätsforsch Allerg Klin Immunol 1959; 118:349–357.
32 Alper CA, Rosen FS: Increased susceptibility to infection in patients with defects affecting C3. Birth Defects 1975;11:301–306.
33 Götze O, Müller-Eberhard HJ: The C3-activator system: An alternate pathway of complement activation. J Exp Med 1971;134:90s–108s.
34 Alper CA, Goodkofsky I, Lepow IH: The relationship of glycine-rich β-glycoprotein to factor B in the properdin system and to the cobra factor-binding protein of human serum. J Exp Med 1973;137:424–437.
35 Abramson N, Alper CA, Lachmann PJ, Rosen FS, Jandl JH: Deficiency of C3 inactivator in man. J Immunol 1971;107:19–27.
36 Alper CA, Rosen FS, Lachmann PJ: Inactivator of the third component of complement as an inhibitor in the properdin pathway. Proc Natl Acad Sci USA 1972;69:2910–2913.
37 Alper CA, Abramson N, Johnston RB Jr, Jandl JH, Rosen FS: Studies in vivo and in vitro on an abnormality in the metabolism of C3 in a patient with increased susceptibility to infection. J Clin Invest 1970;49: 1975–1985.
38 Alper CA, Johnson AM: Immunofixation electrophoresis: A technique for the study of protein polymorphism. Vox Sang 1969;17:445–452.
39 Alper CA, Boenisch T, Watson L: Genetic polymorphism in human glycine-rich beta-glycoprotein. J Exp Med 1972;135:68–80.
40 Carroll MC, Campbell RD, Porter RR: Mapping of steroid 21-hydroxylase genes adjacent to complement component C4 genes in HLA, the major histocompatibility complex in man. Proc Natl Acad Sci USA 1985;82:521–525.
41 Teng YS, Tan SG: Subtyping of properdin factor B (Bf) by isoelectrofocusing. Hum Hered 1982;32:362–366.
42 Geserick G, Patzelt D, Schröder H, Nagai T: Isoelectrofocusing in the study of the Bf system. Existence of two common subtypes of the Bf*F allele. Vox Sang 1983;44:178–182.
43 Siemens I, Bender K, Geserick G, Mauff G, Pulverer G: The BF F subtypes are detectable in the Ba fragment of factor B. Forensic Sci Int 1989;42:279–286.
44 Davrinche C, Abbal M, Clerc M: Molecular characterization of human complement factor B subtypes. Immunogenetics 1990;32:309–312.
45 Jahn I, Mejía JE, Thomas M, Darke C, Schröder H, Geserick G, Hauptmann G: Genomic analysis of the F subtypes of human complement factor B. Eur J Immunogenet 1994;21: 415–419.
46 Allen FH Jr: Linkage of HL-A and GBG. Vox Sang 1974;27:382–384.
47 Fu SM, Kunkel HG, Brusman HP, Allen FH Jr, Fotino M: Evidence for linkage between HL-A histocompatibility genes and those involved in the synthesis of the second component of complement. J Exp Med 1974;140:1108–1111.
48 Raum D, Alper CA, Stein R, Gabbay KH: Genetic marker for insulin-dependent diabetes mellitus. Lancet 1979;i:1208–1210.
49 Hobart MJ, Lachmann PJ, Alper CA: Polymorphism of human C6; in Peeters H (ed): Protides of the Biological Fluids. New York, Pergamon Press, 1975, vol 22, pp 575–580.
50 Simon S, Truedsson L, Marcus-Bagley D, Awdeh Z, Eisenbarth GS, Brink SJ, Yunis EJ, Alper CA: Relationship between protein complotypes and DNA variant haplotypes: Complotype-RFLP constellations (CRC). Hum Immunol 1997; 57:27–36.

51 Alper CA, Raum D, Karp S, Awdeh ZL, Yunis EJ: Serum complement 'supergenes' of the major histocompatibility complex in man (complotypes). Vox Sang 1983;45:62–67.
52 Whitehead AS, Woods DE, Fleischnick E, Chin JE, Yunis EJ, Katz AJ, Gerald PS, Alper CA, Colten HR: DNA polymorphism of the C4 genes: A new marker for analysis of the major histocompatibility complex. N Engl J Med 1984;310:88–91.
53 Bentley DR, Campbell RD, Cross RJ: DNA polymorphism of the C2 locus. Immunogenetics 1985;22: 377–390.
54 Cross SJ, Edwards JH, Bentley DR, Campbell RD: Polymorphism of the C2 and factor B genes. Immunogenetics 1985;21:39–48.
55 Fathallah D, Abbal M, Thomsen M, Cambon-Thomsen A, Campbell RD: A DNA restriction fragment length polymorphism in the complement region of the human MHC shows an absolute correlation with polymorphism of complement factor B (BF) defined by isoelectric focusing. J Immunogenet 1985;12: 321–326.
56 Schneider PM, Carroll MC, Alper CA, Rittner C, Whitehead AS, Yunis EJ, Colten HR: Polymorphism of the human complement C4 and steroid 21-hydroxylase genes. Restriction fragment length polymorphisms revealing structural deletions, homoduplications, and size variants. J Clin Invest 1986;78:650–657.
57 Schneider PM, Rittner C: *Bgl* II restriction fragment length polymorphism of human complement C4A gene coincides with BF*F allele of factor B: Immunogenetics 1988;27: 225–228.

Experimental and Clinical Immunogenetics

Exp Clin Immunogenet 1998;15:213–230

Received: August 27, 1998
Accepted: September 30, 1998

C. Yung Yu

Children's Hospital Research Foundation, and Department of Pediatrics, Department of Medical Microbiology and Immunology, The Ohio State University, Columbus, Ohio, USA

Molecular Genetics of the Human MHC Complement Gene Cluster

Key Words

Complement C4 and C2 deficiencies
Tenascin *TNX*
Steroid 21-hydroxylase *CYP21* and congenital adrenal hyperplasia
Endogenous retrovirus HERV-K(C4)
RCCX modular variation
Unequal crossover
Novel genes *DOM3Z, RD, RP1* and *SKI2W*

Abstract

The human major histocompatibility complex (MHC) complement gene cluster (MCGC) is a highly variable region that is characterized by polymorphisms, variations in gene size and gene number, and associations with diseases. Deficiencies in complement C2 are either due to abolition of C2 protein synthesis by mini-deletions that caused frameshift mutations, or blocked secretion of the C2 protein by single amino acid substitutions. One, two or three *C4* genes may be present in a human MCGC haplotype and these genes may code for C4A, C4B, or both. Deficiencies of C4A or C4B proteins are attributed to the expression of identical *C4* isotypes or allotypes from the *C4* loci, the absence or deletion of a *C4* gene, 2-bp insertion at exon 29 or 1-bp deletion at exon 20 that caused frameshift mutations. The *C4* genes are either 21 or 14.6 kb in size due to the presence of endogenous retrovirus HERV-K(C4) in the intron 9 of long *C4* genes. A deletion or duplication of a *C4* gene is always accompanied by its neighboring genes, *RP* at the 5′ region, and *CYP21* and *TNX* at the 3′ region. These four genes form a genetic unit termed the RCCX module. In an RCCX bimodular structure, the pseudogene *CYP21A*, and partially duplicated gene segments *TNXA* and *RP2* are present between the two *C4* loci. The RCCX modular variations in gene number and gene size contributed to unequal crossovers and exchanges of polymorphic sequences/mutations, resulting in the homogenization of *C4* polymorphisms and acquisitions of deleterious mutations in *RP1, C4A, C4B, CYP21B* and *TNXB* genes. *RD, SKI2W, DOM3Z* and *RP1* are the four novel genes found between *Bf* and *C4*. RD and Ski2w proteins may be related to RNA splicing, RNA turnover and regulation of translation. The functions of Dom3z and RP1 are being investigated. The complete genomic DNA sequence between *C2* and *TNX* is now available. This should facilitate a complete documentation of polymorphisms, mutations and disease associations for the MCGC.

KARGER

Fax + 41 61 306 12 34
E-Mail karger@karger.ch
www.karger.com

Accessible online at:
http://BioMedNet.com/karger

C. Yung Yu
Room W208, Wexner's Institute for Pediatric Research,
700 Children's Drive, Columbus, OH 43205-2696 (USA)
Tel. +1 614 722 2821, Fax +1 614 722 2774
E-Mail cyu@chi.osu.edu

Introduction

The genes coding for subunit proteins of the human complement C3/C5 convertases, C2, factor B (Bf), C4A and C4B are localized in the middle of MHC class III region [1]. The MHC complement gene cluster (MCGC) is defined as the genes located in the genomic region between complement *C2* and extracellular matrix tenascin X *(TNX)*. This gene cluster varies in size from 142 to 214 kb. It is a highly variable genomic region that is characterized by polymorphism, variation in gene size and gene number. Many genetic and immune disorders are associated with the MCGC.

The human MHC (also known as the HLA) is located at the p21.3 region of chromosome 6. The class III region is about 1,100 kb in size and is sandwiched between the class I and II regions [2]. Figure 1 shows a molecular map of the human MCGC. Table 1 lists the data base accession numbers for each gene or gene segment from the MCGC. In the most common haplotype, fourteen genes or gene segments are present in this cluster. Between *Bf* and *C4* are novel genes *RD, SKI2W, DOM3Z* and *RP1.* Downstream of complement *C4A* and *C4B* genes are the steroid 21-hydroxylase A *(CYP21A)* and B *(CYP21B)* genes, respectively. The human *CYP21A* is a pseudogene [3–5]. Overlapping to the 3′ ends of the *CYP21A* and *CYP21B* genes are the tenascin-XA *(TNXA)* and tenascin-XB *(TNXB)* genes, respectively [6]. The gene segment *RP2* is present between *TNXA and C4B* [7]. This review will focus on the genetic instability of the MCGC.

Complement C2 Deficiency

Complement component C2 and factor B provide the essential catalytic subunit of the classical and alternative activation pathway C3/C5 convertases, respectively. The two pro-

Table 1. Genes and gene segments of the HLA complement gene cluster

Genes	Exons	Gene size, kb	Amino acids coded	GenBank accession No.
C2	18	17.9	752	X04481, L09706-8, AF019413
Bf	18	6.0	764	L15702, X72875, AF019413
RD	11	6.7	380	L03411, AF019413
SKI2W	28	10.8	1,246	Z48796, AF059675
DOM3Z	7	2.2	396	AF059252, L26261, AF059675
RP1/G11	9/7	11/9	364/254	L26260, X77386, L26261
C4A	41	21/14.6	1,744	K02403, M59815, U07856, M59816
CYP21A	10	3.2	–	M26857, M12793, M13935
TNXA	13	4.5	–	L26263, U24488
RP2	3	0.9	–	L26263, L26262
C4B	41	21/14.6	1,744	K02404, U24578
CYP21B	10	3.2	495	M26856, M12792, M13936, AF77974
TNXB	45	68.2	4,289	U89337
XB-S	13	4.5	673	U24488, AF077974

teins share 41.7% overall sequence identities or 62.9% sequence similarities [8–10]. Each protein is about 100 kD in size. The *C2* and *Bf* genes are separated by 421 bp [11]. Each gene contains 18 exons but the *C2* gene is three times larger than the *Bf* gene [12] due to the presence of larger introns and a retroposon SVA in intron 3 of the *C2* gene [7, 13]. SVA is a composite retroposon that contains a SINE element, multiple copies of GC-rich variable number tandem repeats (of which each copy is 35–45 bp in size), and an *Alu*

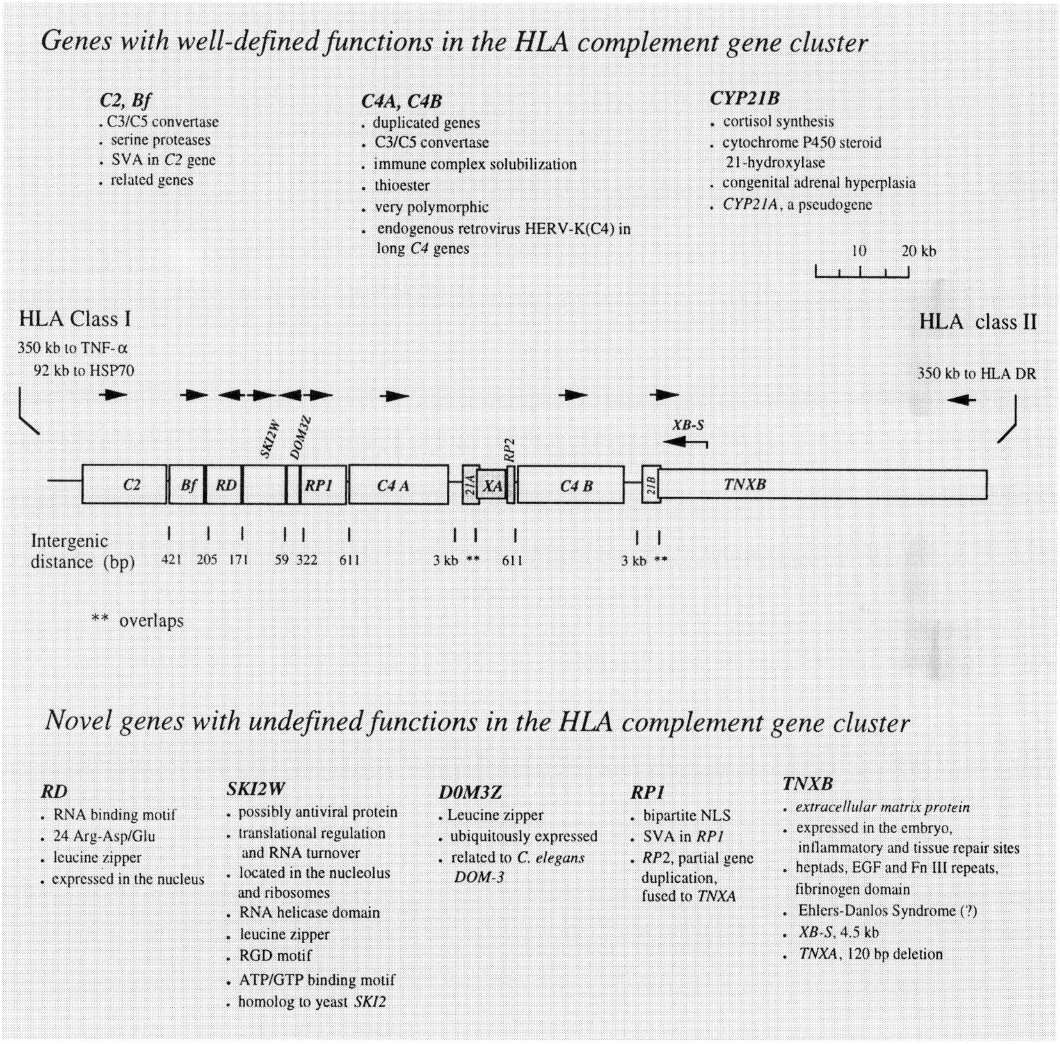

Fig. 1. Organization of the MCGC with a bimodular RCCX structure and features of the genes and gene segments in the MCGC. A horizontal arrow represents the transcriptional configuration. XA = TNXA; 21A = CYP21A; 21B = CYP21B; NLS = nuclear localization signal.

Table 2. Molecular basis of human complement C2 deficiency

Prevalence: 1% Caucasians	
Diseases associated: SLE, glomerulonephritis, vasculitis	
Type I deficiency:	No C2 protein
1 Haplotype:	HLA *A25 B18 DRw2, BfS C2Q0 C4A4 B2*
Defect:	28-bp deletion – 9 bp of exon 6 and 19 bp of intron 6; exon 6 skipped in C2 mRNA, frameshift mutation
2 Haplotype:	HLA *A3 B35 DR4 DQ1, BfF C2Q0 C4A32 BQ0*
Defect:	1-bp deletion at exon 2, frameshift mutation
Type II deficiency:	C2 protein not secreted
1 Haplotype:	HLA *A11 B35 DRw1, BfS C2Q0 C4AQ0 B1*
Mutation:	exon 5, C566T
Substitution:	Ser 189 Phe
2 Haplotype:	HLA *A2 B5 DRw4, C4A3B1*
Mutation:	exon 11, G1930A
Substitution:	Gly 444 Arg
3 Haplotype:	HLA *A28 B58 DR12*
Mutation:	exon 3, G392A
Substitution:	Cys 111 Tyr

element altogether enclosed by direct terminal repeats [7].

Hereditary deficiency of C2 is the commonest form of complement deficiencies. Heterozygous deficiency of C2 is present in about 1% of the Caucasians. The predominant type (type I) of C2 deficiency is present in the HLA haplotype *A25 B18 DR2* and complotype *S042 (Bf-S, C2Q0, C4A4 C4B2)*. The majority of type I C2 deficiency is the result of a 28 bp deletion at the 5′ splice junction at exon 6 of the *C2* gene. This leads to the skipping of exon 6 during RNA splicing and therefore a deletion of 134 bp in the *C2* transcript, resulting in a frame shift mutation and premature termination at the N-terminal domain of the C2 protein [14]. A second cause for the type I deficiency has been found to be a 2-bp deletion in exon 2. This deletion leads to a frame shift and immediate stop codon, resulting in an absence of detectable C2 protein synthesis [15].

About 10% of C2 deficiency belongs to the type II deficiency that is the result of a secretion defect of the C2 protein. Studies on three cases of type II deficiency all pointed to single amino acid substitutions in the C2 protein, which are S189F, G444R, and C111Y [16, 17] (table 2). How do these single amino acid changes block the secretion of C2 remains to be determined.

In contrast to C2 deficiency, deficiency in factor B is rare. A targeted disruption of *Bf* in the mouse also resulted in the loss of expression of two flanking genes, which are the upstream *C2* gene and the downstream *RD* gene in addition to *Bf*. In other words, the resulting mouse is deficient in both alternative and classical pathways of complement activation [18]. It is of interest to investigate the physiological impact of the RD deficiency.

Table 3. Polymorphisms and deficiencies of complement C4

		C4A	C4B
1	Electrophoretic mobility		
	(a) Agarose gel	fast (acidic)	slow (basic)
	(b) SDS-PAGE (α chain)	Mr 96 000	Mr 94 000
2	Thioester reactivity		
	(a) Hemolytic activity	lower	higher
	(b) Relative covalent binding affinities		
	Amino group	higher	lower
	Hydroxyl group	lower	higher
3	Antigenic determinants[1]	Rodgers, WH	Chido, WH
	Blood group antigen	Rg: 1, 2	Ch: 1, 2, 3, 4, 5, 6
4	Defective C5 convertase	C4A6	C4B1(hi)
	Mutation	Arg 458 Trp	Pro 459 Leu
5	Deficiencies		
	Mutation	exon 29, 2-bp insertion	exon 29, 2-bp insertion
	Haplotype	HLA *A2 B40 DR6*	HLA *B39 Cw7*
	Mutation	exon 20, 1-bp deletion	
	Haplotype	HLA *A30 B18 DR3*	

[1] With exceptions such as C4A1 and C4B5.

Structural Variations of Complement C4

Polymorphisms of C4A and C4B

The covalent binding ability through the *thioester* carbonyl group after activation, and the relatively large size with ~ 200 kD, enable C4 to link and provide surfaces for protein interactions among the antigen-antibody complex, complement components C2, C3, C5, regulatory proteins factor I, C4b binding protein, complement receptor type I (CR1), and possibly membrane cofactor protein MCP. C4 is complex both at the protein and the genomic levels (table 3). There are two isotypes of C4, C4A (*a*cidic) and C4B (*b*asic) with more than 34 allotypes altogether [19–21]. The C4A and C4B proteins are markedly different in electrophoretic mobilities, hemolytic activities, and chemical reactivities [22–24]. The latter is due to the differential reactivities of the thioester carbonyl group in the two classes of C4: C4A exhibits 100-fold higher covalent binding affinity to amino groups or peptide antigens than C4B, while C4B binds to hydroxyl groups or carbohydrate antigens 10-fold more efficient than C4A [22, 25]. This difference in reactivity explains why C4A binds to immune complexes three times more effectively than C4B [25, 26]. C4A proteins are usually associated with the Rodgers antigens (Rg1, Rg2). C4B proteins are usually associated with the Chido antigens (Ch1–Ch6) [20, 27].

In both C4A and C4B, protein variants with low hemolytic activities or with reversed association of serologic properties have been found. It has been shown that C4A6 and a

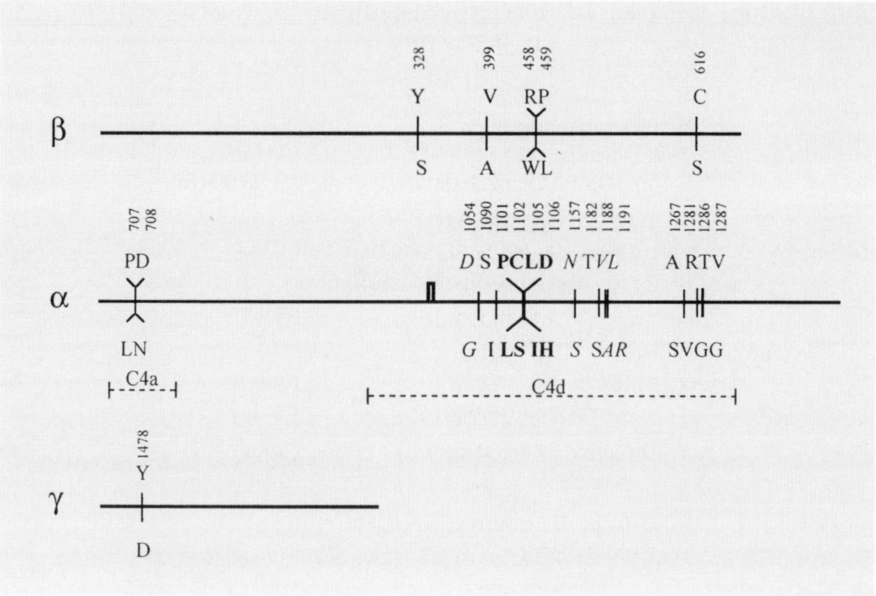

Fig. 2. Polymorphic amino acid residues on C4A and C4B. The thioester bond is shown as an open box. The isotypic residues are in bold, the Rg and Ch antigenic determinants are italicized.

subtype of C4B1, C4B1(hi), are almost *h*emolytically *i*nactive [28–31]. These low hemolytic activities are due to the presence of a defective C5 convertase caused by the Arg_{458} to Trp_{458} substitution for C4A6, and Pro_{459} to Leu_{459} mutation for C4B1(hi). These two mutations are both located on the β-chain [30], suggesting the presence of a C5 binding site in the β-chain of the three-chained (β-α-γ) C4 molecule. The differential chemical reactivities of C4A and C4B are determined by variations of four amino acids at positions 1101–1106, by which C4A has the sequence PCPVLD, while C4B has the sequence LSPVIH [32, 33]. Site-directed mutagenesis experiments further indicated that D1106 for C4A and H1106 for C4B are important in determining the formation of amide bonds and ester bonds, respectively, with the targets [34, 35]. Besides the isotypic differences at residues 1101–1106, D1054G, N1157S, VDLL1188–1191ADLR are common amino acid changes associated with C4A and C4B, respectively, at the C4d region. These amino acid variations constitute the sequential and conformational epitopes for the Rg and Ch antigenic determinants [20, 32]. The C4B isotypic residues are also associated with the Ch4 antigen. Therefore, shuffling of the discrete sequences at 1101–1106 will lead to the reversion of C4A to C4B, or vice versa. Shuffling of the sequences at positions 1054, 1157, 1188–1191 will change the association of the Rg or Ch antigenic determinants with the C4 molecules. The most typical examples are the association of C4A1 with Ch1, 3, 5, 6, and C4B5 with Rg1 and with Ch4 and Ch6 [20, 27, 32]. In addition, the association of S1157 with VDLL1188–1191, in either C4A or C4B, leads to the formation of another conformational epitope WH [36, 37]. The locations of polymorphic residues in C4A and C4B are shown in figure 2.

Variation in the Number of C4 *Genes*

The complexity of *C4* genetics is extraordinary: there is an unusually frequent variation in the number and size of *C4* genes. Through protein allotyping and genetic studies, it was found that 64.5–74.5% of chromosome 6 in the population contains two different *C4* genes, *C4A* and *C4B*, 16–19% contains *C4B* genes only, 9.5–14.5% contains *C4A* genes only, and 1–2% contains three *C4* genes, or two *C4A* genes, or two *C4B* genes [38]. In most cases, there are two tandem *C4* loci. Locus I frequently codes for *C4A* and locus II frequently codes for *C4B*. However, there are examples for the two C4 loci coding for identical C4 isotypes or allotypes from two C4 loci [39–44].

C4A and C4B Deficiencies

Complete deficiencies of C4A and C4B are rare but highly deleterious [38, 45–47]. Almost all complete C4 deficiency patients suffer systemic lupus, discoid lupus, and immune complex disease in the kidney or overwhelming infections. On the contrary, partial and complete deficiencies of either C4A or C4B are common which exist in 10–30% of the Caucasian population [48]. Deficiencies of C4A or C4B can be due to the absence or deletion of a specific *C4A* or *C4B* gene [49], the presence of two genes coding for identical C4 isotypes or allotypes [39, 44], or the presence of pseudogenes caused by mini-deletions or point mutations. The major cause for the nonexpression of a *C4A* gene (i.e. pseudogene) is due to a 2-bp insertion into the exon 29, which causes a premature termination of the C4A protein at the C4d region [50]. This *C4AQ0* pseudogene is most frequently present in HLA haplotype *A2 B40 Cw3* [45, 50]. Such a 2-bp insertion has also been found in a *C4BQ0* gene with the HLA haplotype *A2 B39 Cw7 DRB1*1501, DRB5*0101 DQB1*0602* [51]. A rare single nucleotide deletion has been detected in exon 20 that would generate a premature termination codon; it has been discovered in HLA *A30 B18 F1C00 DR3* [52].

The Long and Short C4 *Genes*

The complete genomic sequences for a *C4A3* gene [53, 54] and two *C4B* genes [55, 56] have been determined. The 5.5-kb coding sequence is split into 41 exons. The C4d region is coded by exons 23 to 30 that span 2.2 kb. The thioester bond, the C4A and C4B isotypic residues, the Rodgers (Rg) and Chido (Ch) antigens and most of the polymorphic sites of C4 are located at the C4d region (fig. 2).

A peculiar feature of the *C4* gene structure is the size dichotomy. When genomic clones for *C4A* and *C4B* genes were mapped for restriction enzyme site patterns, it was found that the *C4A* gene was about 6–7 kb larger than some of the *C4B* genes [1, 32, 57]. The intron 9 for the long *C4* genes is 6.8 kb in size [53, 54]. This intron is only 416 bp in size for the short *C4* gene [54]. When the sequence of the large intron 9 was determined, an endogenous retrovirus, HERV-K(C4), was found [53, 54, 58–60]. HERV-K(C4) contains all the hallmark structures of a retrovirus (fig. 3). These include the 5′ and 3′ long terminal repeats (LTRs) of 548 and 550 bp, respectively. Downstream of the 5′ LTR is the 18 bp, Lys tRNA primer binding site (PBS). Upstream of the 3′ LTR is the 23-bp polypurine track (PPT). The PBS and the PPT are essential structures for retroviral replication. Between the PBS and the PPT are the *gag, pol, env* genes and an AT-rich region. The *gag, pol,* and *env* genes have acquired many point mutations. Therefore, the HERV-K(C4) in the

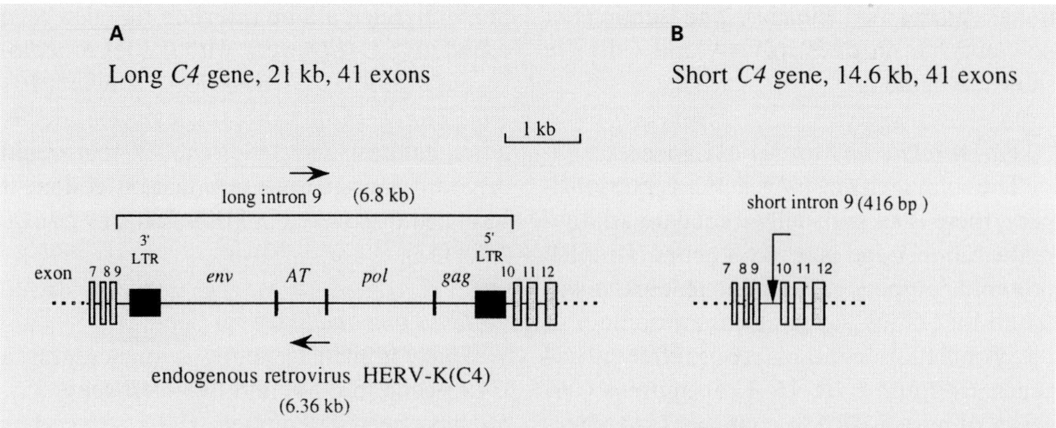

Fig. 3. The size dichotomy of human *C4* genes. **A** Exon-intron structure between exon 7 and exon 12 of a long *C4* gene. A horizontal arrow represents the transcriptional configuration. **B** Exon-intron structure between exon 7 and exon 12 of a short *C4* gene.

C4 gene may not produce a live retrovirus. It is not known, however, whether some of the smaller reading frames would code for superantigens that can stimulate T cell receptors, as it is discussed for insulin-dependent diabetes mellitus (IDDM) and in some other autoimmune diseases [61, 62].

There is a spectrum of haplotypes for the *C4* genes with and without the endogenous retrovirus. In the Caucasian population more than 78.4% of the *C4* genes contain HERV-K(C4) [C. A. Blanchong and C.Y. Yu, unpubl. obs.]. In a duplicated haplotype, the two *C4* genes are mainly long-long (L-L) or long-short (L-S). However, in 2 Caucasians [48] and in certain tribes of the South American population [63], duplicated *C4* haplotypes with short-short (S-S) configuration are also found. For individuals with a single *C4* gene on the chromosome 6, the *C4* gene is either long or short.

HERV-K(C4) is organized in the opposite transcriptional orientation with respect to the *C4* gene. Therefore, transcription of the *C4* gene produces the antisense version for the retrovirus. Such a configuration may have selection advantage for the host because the antisense RNA for HERV-K(C4) could hybridize to proviral genomic RNAs and therefore served as a neutralizing agent to inhibit retroviral proliferations.

Multiple copies of the HERV-K(C4) are present in the human genome [54]. When a genomic DNA probe spanning the LTR and part of the *env* gene was hybridized to a primate zoo blot, about 30–50 restriction fragments were detected in human, orangutan, chimpanzee, gorilla and African green monkey. However, this family of endogenous retroviruses is not present in New World primates such as the cotton-top tamarin, suggesting that the retroviral integration into the *C4* gene occurred shortly after the split between the Old World and the New World primates. While long and short *C4* genes have been found in most nonhuman primates, it is intriguing to note that chimpanzee and gorilla *C4* genes are all short, although family members of the ERV-K(C4) are present in these great apes [58, 64, 65].

The Steroid 21-Hydroxylase Genes *CYP21A* and *CYP21B*

In 1985, the steroid 21-hydroxylase genes *CYP21A* and *CYP21B* were mapped downstream of the complement *C4A* and *C4B* genes [66, 67]. *CYP21* is essential for the biosynthesis of glucocorticoid and mineralocorticoid hormones [68]. Complete absence of *CYP21* leads to salt-wasting, low activity of *CYP21* causes simple virilizing, while below average *CYP21* activity causes androgen excess. *CYP21A* is a pseudogene because it contains three deleterious mutations that include an 8-bp deletion in exon 3, resulting in a frame shift mutation. In addition, there are many point mutations both in coding sequence and in introns [3–5]. If the deleterious mutations of *CYP21A* are incorporated into *CYP21B*, or if the *CYP21B* gene is deleted, in both copies of the chromosome 6, the patient suffers congenital adrenal hyperplasia (CAH).

The Tenascin *TNXA* and *TNXB* Genes Overlap to *CYP21A* and *CYP21B*, Respectively

While characterizing the transcripts of *CYP21* from CAH patients, it was discovered that a pair of duplicated genes, *TNXA* and *TNXB*, *overlap* to the 3′ regions of *CYP21A* and *CYP21B*, respectively. The transcriptional orientations of *TNXA and TNXB* are opposite to those of *CYP21* and *C4* [6, 69].

The duplication of *TNX* is incomplete. Structural characterization revealed that the *TNXB* gene is 68.2 kb in size, consists of 45 exons and codes for a transcript ~13 kb in size [70–72]. Derived amino acid sequence of TNXB reveals a heptad, 18.5 epidermal growth factor repeats, thirty-two fibronectin type III (Fn III) repeats and a fibrinogen domain. Each subunit of TNX protein may be >500 kD in size. However, a smaller transcript about 2.6 kb in size related to *TNX* has also been detected and cloned. This transcript arises from a cryptic promoter site within intron 32 of the *TNXB* gene [73]. This smaller gene is designated *XB-S*. The *XB-S* transcript is expressed only in the adrenal gland. It encodes a 74-kD protein that is identical to the carboxyl 673 residues of TNXB. It contains five fibronectin type-III-like repeats and the carboxyl terminal fibrinogen domain. The function of XB-S is unknown but is suggested to be an evolutionary precursor to the tenascin protein family.

TNXA appears to be a partially duplicated gene segment that corresponds to intron 32 to exons 45 of the *TNXB*. *TNXA* is virtually identical to *XB-S* except for the presence of a 120-bp deletion, of which 91 bp is present in exon 36. This deletion results in a frame shift mutation and premature termination of translation [7, 74].

The function of *TNXB* has not been defined, but its transcripts are ubiquitously expressed in the fetus, with highest levels detectable in muscle and testis [70]. The overall structure of *TNXB* shows striking similarities to extracellular matrix protein, tenascin-related molecules cytostatin (TN-C) and restrictin (TN-R) [75]. Immunochemical and immunohistochemical analyses of the mouse and rat TNX proteins revealed prominent expression in the extracellular matrix surrounding muscle cells of skeletal muscles and cardiac muscles. TNX proteins were also detectable in skin, developing digestive tract, blood vessels and in a renal carcinoma cell line [72, 76, 77]. It has been suggested that deficiency of TNX is associated with the Ehlers-Danlos syndrome (EDS), which is characterized by connective tissue disorder and poor wound healing [78].

Other *CYP21* and *C4*-Related Transcripts in Adrenals

Analyses of *CYP21*- and *C4*-related transcripts in adrenals yielded further tantalizing observations. First, *CYP21A*- and *CYP21B*-related transcripts, designated *YA* and *YB* are present in great abundance in adrenal RNA [79]. *YA* appeared to be a partially spliced *CYP21A* transcript at the 5′ region but continued to the sequence complementary to *TNXA*, and probably ended at the *RP2* genomic region. *YB* appears to be a partially spliced transcript for *CYP21B* that continued to sequence complementary to *TNXB*. No protein products for the *YA* and *YB* transcripts, which have both 7.5- and 3-kb isoforms, have been reported because their reading frames are closed. Therefore, the significance of these Y-transcripts remains to be elucidated. Second, a 1-kb transcript corresponding to exon 35–41 of complement *C4A* and *C4B* genes was detected in RNAs isolated from fetal and adult adrenal cortex. Such transcript could produce a 15-kD polypeptide that is similar to the carboxyl terminal region of the C4 γ-chain. However, no endogenous protein product for this 1-kb transcript has been detected and its putative protein product generated by in vitro translation did not cross-react with C4 antisera [80].

RP1 and *RP2* Are Present Upstream of Complement *C4A* and *C4B*, Respectively

RP1 (also known as G11) and *RP2* are located 611 bp upstream of the human *C4A* and *C4B* genes, respectively. The putative RP1/G11 protein, consists of 364 or 258 amino acid residues [7, 81]. The difference is attributable to variations at the 5′ regions of transcripts in the two reports. The larger transcript extends the reading frame by 106 amino acids. However, this extended sequence is not conserved in mouse RP1 [Yang Z. et al., in preparation]. Determination of the N-terminal sequence from the endogenous RP1 protein would settle the discrepancy. The function of RP1 is unknown. The deduced protein sequence is basic and hydrophilic. There is a bipartite nuclear localization signal and therefore RP1 may be a nuclear protein. Northern blot analysis suggested that *RP1* is ubiquitously expressed.

The *RP1* gene contains nine exons (or seven exons for the smaller, G11 gene/transcript). Located in the fourth intron is a cluster of *Alu* elements, and a newly defined composite retroposon SVA. Members of SVA are also present in the complement *C2* gene located about 20 kb upstream of *RP1* in the HLA [82].

Similar to *TNX, RP* is partially duplicated. The duplicated gene segment *RP2* is identical to the last 913 bp of the *RP1* gene and is unlikely to code for a gene product. The gene segments *RP2* and *TNXA* form a chimeric structure between *CYP21A* and *C4B*. Determination of the DNA sequences for *RP2* from two different HLA haplotypes revealed that the identical hybrid sequences resulted from the fusion of the 3′ regions of *RP* and *TNX* genes.

Modular Variations of *RP-C4-CYP21-TNX* (RCCX)

The four tandemly arranged genes *RP*, complement *C4*, steroid 21-hydroxylase *(CYP21)*, and tenascin *TNX* appear to be organized as a genetic unit designated as an RCCX module. Deletions or duplications of *C4* genes are always accompanied by their neighboring genes in the RCCX, i.e., *RP, CYP21* and *TNX* [7, 83–85]. Duplication or

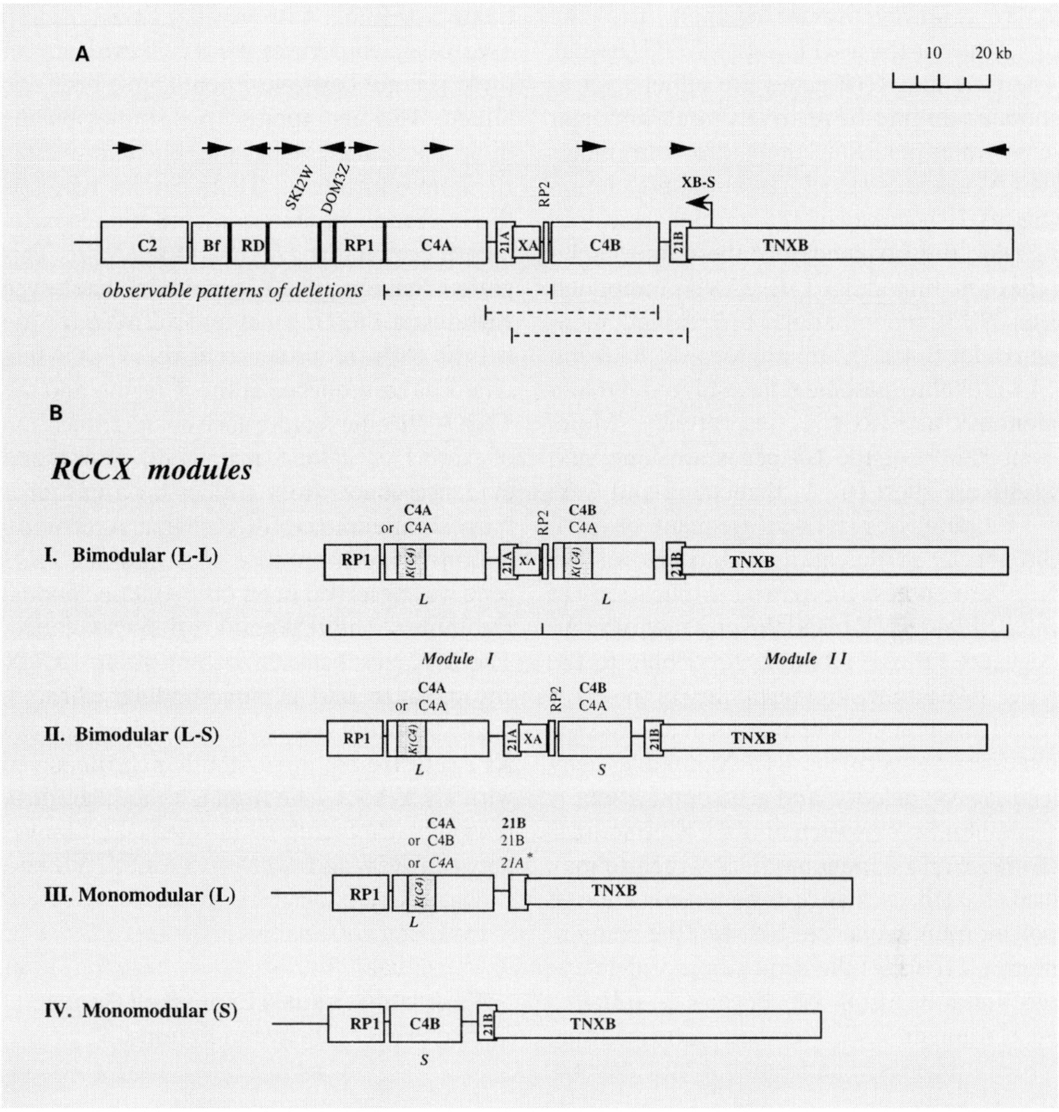

Fig. 4. RCCX modular variations. **A** Observable patterns of gene deletions in the MCGC. Arrows represent transcriptional orientations. **B** RCCX haplotypes. K(C4), endogenous retrovirus HERV-K(C4). The common C4 and CYP21 haplotypes are in bold. An asterisk indicates the haplotype is associated with CAH.

triplication of the RCCX modules occurred by the addition of a genomic segment of either 32.5 or 26.2 kb containing a long or a short *C4* gene, a *CYP21* gene together with the *TNXA-RP2* chimera. In an RCCX bimodular haplotype, the three genes/ gene segments present between the two *C4* loci, *CYP21A, TNXA* and *RP2* are all corrupted sequences with no obvious functional products. In an RCCX monomodular haplotype, the intact genes *RP1* and

TNXB are always present together with a *C4A* or *C4B* gene, and a *CYP21A* or *CYP21B* gene. The *C4A* and *C4B* genes are either long or short. Excluding the relatively rare trimodular haplotypes [21, 86], there are four major RCCX modular structures in the population (fig. 4). In a survey of 128 normal Caucasian females, the frequencies of these four haplotypes are: bimodular L-L, 55.9%; bimodular L-S, 29.7%; monomodular L, 3.5% and, monomodular S, 10.7%. In other words, 85.6 and 14.4% of chromosome 6 have bimodular and monomodular RCCX, respectively. Moreover, 78.4% of the *C4* genes are long, and 21.6% are short [C. A. Blanchong and C.Y. Yu, unpubl. obs.]. These frequent physical differences in the number and size of the RCCX modules, the partial duplications of the *RP2* and *TNXA*, and the presence of pseudogene *CYP21A*, probably contribute to the genetic variability and instability of the HLA class III region. Misalignments of and recombinations between the RCCX modules may lead to gene deletion and gene duplication. A recombination between an RCCX bimodular structure and a monomodular structure may lead to (1) the exchange or homogenization of polymorphic sequences between the complement *C4* loci, (2) the acquisition of deleterious mutations from pseudogene *CYP21A* or gene segment *TNXA* to their corresponding structural genes. The former is best demonstrated by the presence of the C4A-associated amino acid residues in many C4B allotypes, and vice versa. The latter is manifested in many disease-associated haplotypes such as the acquisition of the 2-bp insertion in exon 29 from *C4AQ0* to *C4BQ0* in a SLE patient [51], the presence of a *CYP21A/CYP21B* hybrid gene in the HLA B47 *C4A1* haplotype of CAH patients [87, 88], and the presence of a *TNXB/TNXA* hybrid gene with the 120-bp mini-deletion in conjunction with the deletion of the *RP2-C4B-CYP21B* gene in patients with CAH and possibly EDS [78, 89]. Two other important pieces of evidence of these genetic crossover events have been obtained. The first comes from studies on the molecular genetics of a pauciarticular juvenile rheumatoid arthritis (JRA) patient who has the reciprocal product for a genetic recombination between a *TNXA* and a *TNXB*. This patient has an RCCX bimodular haplotype with two *CYP21B* genes and a *TNXB/TNXA* hybrid with the presence of the TNXB-specific 120-bp sequence at the 3′ region and the TNXA-specific feature such as the truncation of exons 1–32 at the 5′ region [90]. The second evidence comes from studies on a nasopharyngeal carcinoma (NPC) cell line. A recombination between an *RP1* gene and a *CYP21* gene was observed in an NPC cell line and its recombination breakpoint region was cloned. The synapsis between a bimodular RCCX chromosome and a monomodular chromosome probably led to the alignment of the *RP1* gene from a monomodular chromosome with a *CYP21A* gene from a bimodular chromosome and therefore an unequal crossover between *RP1* and *CYP21* [89, C.Y. Yu and colleagues, unpubl. obs.].

Four Ubiquitously Expressed Genes Are Present Between *Bf* and *C4*

In the 30 kb genomic segment between *Bf* and *C4* are novel genes *RD-SKI2W-DOM3Z-RP1* whose functions are yet to be determined. *RD*, which codes for a putative RNA binding protein, is 205 bp downstream of *Bf* [71]. The *RD* gene is 6.7 kb in size, consists of eleven exons and is organized in a tail-to-tail configuration with *Bf*. The putative RD protein has 380 amino acids [91–93]. It contains the RNA recognition motif (RRM) of the ribonucleoprotein family. However, the most striking feature of RD is the presence of twenty-four copies of alternate, positively and negatively charged residues, Arg-Asp (RD) [94], which may be related to RNA binding. The cellular function of RD has not been determined.

SKI2W, a DEVH-box gene probably involved in RNA turnover, is 171 bp downstream of *RD*. The *SKI2W* gene consists of 28 exons that produces a 4.0-kb transcript and encodes a polypeptide of 1,246 amino acids. The Ski2w protein contains an RNA helicase domain, two leucine zipper motifs that may be involved in protein-protein interaction, and an RGD motif that may be a ligand for cell adhesion molecules. Indirect immunofluorescence experiments showed that Ski2w is present in the nucleolus and also in the cytoplasm [95]. Immunoblot analysis further revealed that in the cytoplasm of HeLa cell extracts, Ski2w associates with ribosomes and polyribosomes [95]. ATPase activities were demonstrated from fusion proteins containing human Ski2w [96]. Hydrolysis of ATP is required as an energy source for helicases to unwind helical structures of nucleic acids [97]. The human Ski2w protein shares extensive sequence similarity to the yeast antiviral protein Ski2p. Ski2p probably has a general role on the RNA turnover or the regulation of RNA degradation [98–100]. Studies using yeast *ski2* mutants inferred that Ski2p inhibits translation of poly(A)$^-$ RNAs, and interacts with exosomes on the 3′ to 5′ exoribonuclease degradation of RNA molecules. It is proposed that human Ski2w plays a role on linking the polysomes and exosomes together to achieve one of the crucial steps on the temporal control of gene expression, i.e., to facilitate the degradation of mRNAs and to prohibit the degrading mRNAs from being translated [95].

Fifty-nine base-pairs downstream of *SKI2W* is *DOM3Z*. The human *DOM3Z* gene is 2.2 kb in size that contains 7 exons. The 1.4 kb *DOM3Z* transcripts are present in all tissues but higher levels of expression were detected in reproductive tissues and pancreas. The derived amino acid sequence for Dom3z has 396 amino acids that contains a leucine zipper motif and is relatively rich in proline and leucine residues [101]. Dom3z-related proteins are present in simple and complex eukaryotes. In *Caenorhabditis elegans*, Dom3z- related protein could be involved in the development of germ cells [102]. The function of human Dom3z is being investigated.

RD-SKI2W and *DOM3Z-RP1* are arranged as two head-to-head orientated gene pairs separated by only 59 nucleotides. Both gene pairs have unmethylated CpG sequences at the common 5′ regulatory region. The ubiquitous expression pattern suggested that these four genes are probably housekeeping genes [83, 101].

Ski2w and Dom3z have related sequences present in simple and complex eukaryotes. The RNA binding motif present in RD is a conserved protein domain in eukaryotes. RP1 is the only protein among the four novel proteins whose genes are located between *Bf* and *C4* that has not been shown to contain a distinct protein domain present in simple organisms. The tight linkage of *RD, SKI2W, DOM3Z* and *RP*, the ubiquitous gene expression pattern, the presence of leucine zipper motifs in RD, Ski2w and Dom3z, and the potential to bind RNAs (for RD and Ski2w) imply that these proteins may have concerted functions, possibly related to RNA translation and turnover. Genetic and functional studies of these four ubiquitously expressed genes may help elucidate the molecular basis of disease associations with the HLA complement gene cluster.

Conclusions

Every gene or gene segment in the human MCGC has been sequenced by individual laboratories (table 1). However, a complete sequence of 148,855 bp spanning from complement C2 to *TNXB* of a monomodular RCCX/C4B-long haplotype has become available, thanks to the human genome project [55, 71]. This valuable sequence allows the analysis of the regulatory sequences, the presence of all repetitive DNA or mobile genetic elements. It gives a framework for the mapping of polymorphic sites and mutations in the MCGC. It is now feasible to determine sequences for all polymorphic variants of the MCGC genes, particularly the very polymorphic *C4A* and *C4B*. To accommodate all sequence data and to make it available to the public, a mutation database may be created on the internet. Meanwhile, convenient DNA typing techniques for C4, C2 and Bf would be developed and applied in parallel with HLA typing (for C4 and Bf see reference typing reports in this issue [103, 104]). This information will prove valuable for HLA haplotype matching, for forensic purposes and for anthropologic studies. The complete sequence of the 1,100-kb MHC class III region is expected to be completed soon and most, if not all, transcriptional units (novel genes) will be elucidated. The availability of the expressed sequence tag (EST) clones from the IMAGE Consortium [105] will allow a jump-start for studies on functional genomics by circumventing the tedious, initial screening and cloning processes. The major challenge will be to elucidate the physiological functions of the novel genes and connect them with some of the HLA associated diseases.

Acknowledgments

I am indebted to my present and past colleagues, Carol A. Blanchong, Xiaodong Qu, Kristi L. Rupert, Zhenyu Yang, Bi Zhou, Bradley J.Baker, Andrew W. Dangel, Anna R. Mendoza, Audra J. Parker, Salih Sanlioglu, Liming Shen and Shanxiang Zhang who contributed experimental data for this review, and Allyson Amann for secretarial assistance. This work was supported by grants from NIAMSD, National Institutes of Health (R01 AR43969), the Children's Hospital Research Foundation, Columbus Ohio (210698), the March of Dimes Birth Defects Foundation (FY95-1087, Basil O'Conner Starter Scholar Research Award), American Cancer Society- Ohio Division, and the Pittsburgh Supercomputing Center through the NIH Center for Research Resources Cooperative Agreement (1P41 RR06009).

References

1 Carroll MC, Campbell RD, Bentley DR, Porter RR: A molecular map of the human major histocompatibility complex class III region linking complement genes C4, C2 and factor B. Nature 1984;307:237–241.
2 Aguado BMCM,Campbell RD: Genes of the MHC class III region and the functions of the proteins hey encode; in Browning M, McMichael A (eds): HLA and MHC: Genes, Molecules and Function. Oxford, BIOS Scientific Publishers, 1996, pp 39–75.
3 Higashi Y, Yoshioka H, Yamane M, Gotoh O, Fujii-Kuriyama Y: Complete nucleotide sequence of two steroid 21-hydroxylase genes tandemly arranged in human chromosome: A pseudogene and a genuine gene. Proc Natl Acad Sci USA 1986;83: 2841–2845.
4 White PC, New MI, DuPont B: Structure of human steroid 21-hydroxylase genes. Proc Natl Acad Sci USA 1986;83:5111–5115.
5 Rodrigues NR, Dunham I, Yu CY, Carroll MC, Porter RR, Campbell RD: Molecular characterization of the HLA-linked steroid 21-hydroxylase B gene from an individual with congenital adrenal hyperplasia. EMBO J 1987;6:1653–1661.
6 Morel Y, Bristow J, Gitelman SE, Miller WL: Transcript encoded on the opposite strand of the human steroid 21-hydroxylase/complement component C4 gene locus. Proc Natl Acad Sci USA 1989;86: 6582–6586.

7 Shen LM, Wu LC, Sanlioglu S, Chen R, Mendoza AR, Dangel A, Carroll MC, Zipf W, Yu CY: Structure and genetics of the partially duplicated gene RP located immediately upstream of the complement C4A and C4B genes in the HLA class III region: Molecular cloning, exon-intron structure, composite retroposon and breakpoint of gene duplication. J Biol Chem 1994;269:8466–8476.

8 Bentley DR: Primary structure of human complement component C2: Homology to two unrelated protein families. Biochem J 1986;239:339–345.

9 Gagnon J: Structure and activation of complement C2 and factor B. Phil Trans R Soc 1984;306:301–309.

10 Campbell RD, Bentley DR, Morley BJ: The factor B and C2 genes. Phil Trans R Soc Lond 1984;B306:367–378.

11 Wu L-C, Morley BJ, Campbell RD: Cell-specific expression of the human complement protein factor B gene: Evidence for the role of two distinct 5′-flanking elements. Cell 1987;48:331–342.

12 Yoshitomo I, Zeng-Bian Z, Macon K, Volanakis J: Structure of the human C2 gene. J Immunol 1993;151: 170–174.

13 Zhu Z-B, Jian B, Volanakis J: Ancestry of SINE-R.C2 a human-specific retroposon. Hum Genet 1994; 93:545–551.

14 Johnson CA, Densen P, Hurford RK Jr, Colten HR, Wetsel RA: Type I human complement C2 deficiency. J Biol Chem 1992;267:9347–9353.

15 Wang X, Circolo A, Lokki ML, Shackelford PG, Wetsel RA, Colten HR: Molecular heterogeneity in deficiency of complement protein C2 type I. Immunology 1998;93:184–191.

16 Wetsel RA, Kulics J, Lokki ML, Kiepiela P, Akama H, Johnson CA, Densen P, Colten HR: Type II human complement C2 deficiency. Allele-specific amino acid substitutions (Ser189 → Phe; Gly444 → Arg) cause impaired C2 secretion. J Biol Chem 1996;271:5824–5831.

17 Zhu ZB, Atkinson TP, Volanakis JE: A novel type II complement C2 deficiency allele in an African-American family. J Immunol 1998; 161:578–584.

18 Taylor PR, Nash JT, Theodoridis E, Bygrave AE, Walport MJ, Botto M: A targeted disruption of the murine complement factor B gene resulting in loss of expression of three genes in close proximity, factor B, C2 and D17H6S45. J Biol Chem 1998;273: 1699–1704.

19 Mauff G, Alper CA, Dawkins R, Doxiadis G, Giles CM, Hauptmann G, Rittner C, Schneider PM: C4 nomenclature statement (1990). Complement Inflamm 1990;7:261–268.

20 Yu CY, Campbell RD, Porter RR: A structural model for the location of the Rodgers and the Chido antigenic determinants and their correlation with the human complement C4A/C4B isotypes. Immunogenetics 1988;27:399–405.

21 Mauff G, Brenden M, Braun-Stilwell M, Doxiadis G, Giles CM, Hauptmann G, Rittner C, Schneider PM, Stradmann-Bellinghausen B, Uring-Lambert B: C4 reference typing report. Complement Inflamm 1990;7:193–212.

22 Isenman D, Young JR: The molecular basis for the differences in immune hemolysis activity of the Chido and Rodgers isotypes of human complement component C4. J Immunol 1984;132:3019–3027.

23 Isenman DE, Young JR: Covalent binding properties of the CR1 and C4B isotypes of the fourth component of human complement on several C1-bearing cell surfaces. J Immunol 1986;136:2542–2550.

24 Dodds AW, Law S-KA, Porter RR: The purification and properties of some less common allotypes of the fourth component of human complement. Immunogenetics 1986;24: 279–285.

25 Law SKA, Dodds AW, Porter RR: A comparison of the properties of two classes, C4A and C4B, of the human complement component C4. EMBO J 1984;3:1819–1823.

26 Schifferli JA, Hauptmann G, Paccaud J-P: Complement-mediated adherence of immune complexes to human erythrocytes. FEBS Lett 1987;213:415–418.

27 Giles CM, Uring-Lambert B, Goetz J, Hauptmann G, Fielder AHL, Ollier W, Rittner C, Robson T: Antigenic determinants expressed by human C4 allotypes: A study of 325 families provides evidence for the structural antigenic model. Immunogenetics 1988;27:442–448.

28 Dodds AW, Law SK, Porter RR: The origin of the very variable haemolytic activities of the common human complement component C4 allotypes including C4-A6. EMBO J 1985;4:2239–2244.

29 Ebanks RO, Jaikaran ASI, Carroll MC, Anderson MJ, Campbell RD, Isenman DE: A single arginine to tryptophan interchange at β-chain residue 458 of human complement component C4 accounts for the defect in classical pathway C5 convertase activity of allotype C4A6. J Immunol 1992;148:2803–2811.

30 Anderson MJ, Milner CM, Cotton RGH, Campbell RD: The coding sequence of the hemolytically inactive C4A6 allotype of human complement component C4 reveals that a single arginine to tryptophan substitution at β-chain residue 458 is the likely cause of the defect. J Immunol 1992;148:2795–2802.

31 McLean RH, Niblack G, Julian B, Wang T, Wyatt R, Philips III JA, Collins TS, Wickelstein J, Valle D: Hemolytically inactive C4B complement allotype caused by a proline to leucine mutation in the C5-binding site. J Biol Chem 1994;269:27727–27731.

32 Yu CY, Belt KT, Giles CM, Campbell RD, Porter RR: Structural basis of the polymorphism of human complement component C4A and C4B: gene size, reactivity and antigenicity. EMBO J 1986;5:2873–2881.

33 Belt KT, Yu CY, Carroll MC, Porter RR: Polymorphism of human complement component C4. Immunogenetics 1985;21:173–180.

34 Carroll MC, Fathallah DM, Bergamaschini L, Alicot EM, Isenman DE: Substitution of a single amino acid (aspartic acid for histidine) converts the functional activity of human complement C4B to C4A. Proc Natl Acad Sci USA 1990;87:6868–6872.

35 Dodds AW, Ren X-D, Willis AC, Law SKA: The reaction mechanism of the internal thioester in the human complement component C4. Nature 1996;379:177–179.
36 Giles CM: C4: Rodgers and chido typing. Complement Inflamm 1990; 7:213–217.
37 Moulds JM, Roberts Sl, Wells TD: DNA sequence analysis of the C4 antigen WH: Evidence for two mechanisms of expression. Immunogenetics 1996;44:104–107.
38 Hauptmann G, Tappeiner G, Schifferli J: Inherited deficiency of the fourth component of human complement. Immunodeficiency Rev 1988;1:3–22.
39 Yu CY, Campbell RD: Definitive RFLPs to distinguish between the human complement C4A/C4B isotypes and the major Rodgers/Chido determinants: Application to the study of C4 null alleles. Immunogenetics 1987;25:384–390.
40 Palsdottir A, Arnason A, Fossdal R, Jensson O: Gene organization of haplotypes expressing two different C4A allotypes. Hum Genet 1987;76: 220–224.
41 Giles CM, Uring-Lambert B, Boksch W, Braun M, Goetz J, Neumann R, Mauff G, Hauptmann G: The study of a French family with two duplicated C4A haplotypes. Hum Genet 1987;77:359–365.
42 McLean RH, Donohoue PA, Jospe N, Bias WB, Van Dop C, Migeon CJ: Restriction fragment analysis of duplication of the fourth component of complement (C4A). Genomics 1988;2:76–85.
43 McLean RH, Giles CM, Yu CY, Campbell RD, Bias WB: Reversed restriction sites for the C4 isotype and Rodgers (1)/Chido (1) regions on two unique C4 genes. Tissue Antigens 1990;35:75–81.
44 Braun L, Schneider PM, Giles CM, Bertrams J, Rittner C: Null alleles of human complement C4. Evidence for pseudogenes at the C4A locus and for gene conversion at the C4B locus. J Exp Med 1990;171:129–140.
45 Nordin FG, Truedsson L, Sjoholm AG, Kjellman M: DNA analysis in a MHC heterozygous patient with complete C4 deficiency – homozygosity for C4 gene deletion and C4 pseudogene. Exp Clin Immunogenet 1991;8:29–37.
46 Uring-Lambert B, Mascart-Lemone F, Tongio M-M, Goetz J, Hauptmann G: Molecular basis of complete C4 deficiency. A study of three patients. Hum Immunol 1989;24: 125–132.
47 Lokki M-L, Colten HR: Genetic deficiencies of complement. Ann Med 1995;27:451–459.
48 Schneider PM: C4 DNA RFLP reference typing report. Complement Inflamm 1990;7:218–224.
49 Carroll MC, Palsdottir A, Belt KT, Porter RR: Deletion of complement C4 and steroid 21-hydroxylase genes in the HLA class III region. EMBO J 1985;4:2547–2552.
50 Barba G, Rittner C, Schneider PM: Genetic basis of human complement C4A Deficiency: Detection of a point mutation leading to nonexpression. J Clin Invest 1993;91: 1681–1686.
51 Lokki M-L, Circolo A, Ahokas P, Rupert KL, Yu CY, Colten HR: Deficiency of complement protein C4 due to identical frameshift mutations in the *C4A* and *C4B* genes. J Immunol, submitted.
52 Fredrikson GN, Gullstrand B, Schneider PM, Witzel-Schlomp K, Sjoholm AG, Alper CA, Awdeh Z, Truedsson L: Characterization of non-expressed C4 genes in a case of complete C4 deficiency: Identification of a novel point mutation leading to a premature stop codon. Hum Immunol 1998;59:713–719.
53 Yu CY: The complete exon-intron structure of a human complement component C4A gene: DNA sequences, polymorphism, and linkage to the 21-hydroxylase genes. J Immunol 1991;146:1057–1066.
54 Dangel AW, Mendoza AR, Baker BJ, Daniel CM, Carroll MC, Wu L-C, Yu CY: The dichotomous size variation of human complement C4 gene is mediated by a novel family of endogenous retroviruses which also establishes species-specific genomic patterns among Old World primates. Immunogenetics 1994;40: 425–436.
55 Rowen L, Dankers C, Baskin D, Faust J, Loretz C, Ahearn ME, Banta A, Schwartzell S, Smith TM, Spies T, Hood L: *Homo sapiens* HLA class III region containing tenascin X gene, partial cds, cytochrome P450 21-hydroxylase (CYP21B), complement C4 (C4B), G11, helicase (SKI2W), RD, complement factor B (Bf), and complement coomponent C2 (C2) genes, complete cds. GenBank, 1997; Accession no. AF019413.
56 Ulgiati D, Abraham LJ: Comparative analysis of the disease-associated complement C4 gene from the HLA- A1, B8, DR3 haplotype. Exp Clin Immunogenet 1996;13:43–54.
57 Prentice HL, Schneider PM, Strominger JL: C4B gene polymorphism detected in a human cosmid clone. Immunogenetics 1986;23:274–276.
58 Dangel AW, Baker BJ, Mendoza AR, Yu CY: Complement component C4 gene intron 9 as a phylogenetic marker for primates: Long terminal repeats of the endogenous retrovirus ERV-K(C4) are a molecular clock of evolution. Immunogenetics 1995;42:41–52.
59 Chu X, Rittner C, Schneider PM: Length polymorphism of the human compleemnt component C4 gene is due to an ancient retroviral integration. Exp Clin Immunogenet 1995; 12:74–81.
60 Tassabehji M, Strachan T, Anderson M, Campbell RD, Collier S, Lako M: Identification of a novel family of human endogenous retroviruses and characterization of one family member, HERV-K(C4), located in the complement C4 gene cluster. Nucleic Acids Res 1994;22: 5211–5217.
61 Conrad B, Weissmahr RN, Boni R, Arcar J, Schupbach J, Mach B: A human endogenous retroviral superantigen as candidate gene in type I diabetes. Cell 1997;90:303–313.
62 Nakagawa K, Harrison L: The potential roles of endogenous retroviruses in autoimmunity. Immunol Rev 1996;152:193–236.
63 Weg-Remers S, Brenden M, Schwarz E, Witzel K, Schneider PM, Guerra LK, Rehfeldt IR, Lima MT, Hartmann D, Petzl-Erler ML, Messias IJd, Mauff G: Major histocompatibility complex (MHC) class III genetics in two Amerindian tribes from southern Brazil: The Kaingang and the Guarani. Hum Genet 1997;100:548–556.

64 Kawaguchi H, Golubic M, Figueroa F, Klein J: Organization of the chimpanzee *C4-CYP21* region: Implications for the evolution of human genes. Eur J Immunol 1990;20: 739–745.
65 Zhang WJ, Christiansen FT, Wu X, Abraham LJ, Giphart M, Dawkins RL: Organization and evolution of C4 and CYP21 genes in primates: Importance of genomic segments. Immunogenetics 1993;37:170–176.
66 White PC, Grossberger D, Onufer BJ, New MI, DuPont B, Strominger J: Two genes encoding steroid 21-hydroxylase are located near the genes encoding the fourth component of complement in man. Proc Natl Acad Sci USA 1985;82:1089–1093.
67 Carroll MC, Campbell RD, Porter RR: Mapping of steriod 21-hydroxylase genes adjacent to complement C4 genes in HLA, the major histocompatibility complex in man. Proc Natl Acad Sci USA 1985;82:521–525.
68 Miller WL, Morel Y: The molecular genetics of 21-hydroxylase deficiency. Annu Rev Genet 1989;23:371–393.
69 Matsumoto K, Ishihara N, Ando A, Inoko H, Ikemura T: Extracellular matrix protein tenascin-like gene found in human MHC class III region. Immunogenetics 1992;36: 400–403.
70 Bristow J, Tee MK, Gitelman SE, Mellon SH, Miller WL: Tenascin-X: A novel extracellular matrix protein encoded by the human XB gene overlapping P450c21B. J Cell Biol 1993;122:265–278.
71 Rowen L, Dankers C, Baskin D, Faust J, Loretz C, Ahearn ME, Banta A, Schwartzell S, Smith TM, Spies T, Hood L: Human HLA class III region containing cAMP response element binding protein-related protein (CREB-RP) and tenascin-X genes, complete cds, complete sequence. GenBank, 1997;Accession number:U89337.
72 Matsumoto K, Saga Y, Ikemura T, Sakakura T, Chiquet-Ehrishmann R: The distribution of tenascin-X is distinct and often reciprocal to that of tenascin-C. J Cell Biol 1994;125: 483–493.
73 Tee MK, Thomson AA, Bristow J, Miller WL: Sequences promoting the transcription of the human XA gene overlapping P450c21A correctly predict the presence of a novel, adrenal-specific, truncated form of tenascin-X. Genomics 1995;28: 171–178.
74 Gitelman SE, Bristow J, Miller WL: Mechanism and consequences of the duplication of the human C4/ P450c21/gene X locus. Mol Cell Biol 1992;12:2124–2134.
75 Chiquet-Ehrishmann R: Tenascins, a growing family of extracellular matrix proteins. Experientia 1995;51: 853–862.
76 Burch GH, Bedolli MA, McDonough S, Rosenthal SM, Bristow J: Embryonic expression of tenascin-X suggests a role in limb, muscle, and heart development. Dev Dynamics 1995;203:491–504.
77 Geffrotin C, Garrido JJ, Tremet L, Vaiman M: Distinct tissue distribution in pigs of tenascin-X and tenascin- C transcripts. Eur J Biochem 1995;231:83–92.
78 Burch GH, Gong Y, Liu W, Dettman R, Curry CJ, Smith L, Miller WL, Bristow J: Tenascin-X deficiency is associated with Ehlers-Danlos syndrome. Nat Genet 1997;17:104–108.
79 Bristow J, Gitelman SE, Tee MK, Staels B, Miller WL: Abundant adrenal-specific transcription of the human P450c21A 'pseudogene'. J Biol Chem 1993;268:12919–12924.
80 Tee MK, Babalola GO, Aza-Blanc P, Speek M, Gitelman SE, Miller WL: A promoter within intron 35 of the human C4A gene initiates abundant adrenal-specific transcription of a 1 kb RNA: Location of a cryptic CYP21 promoter element? Hum Molec Genet 1995;4:2109–2116.
81 Sargent CA, Anderson MJ, Hsieh A-L, Kendall E, Gomez-Escobar N, Campbell RD: Characterisation of the novel gene G11 lying adjacent to the complement C4A gene in the human major histocompatibility complex. Hum Mol Genet 1994;3:481–488.
82 Zhu ZB, Hsieh S-L, Bentley DR, Campbell RD, Volanakis JE: A variable number of tandem repeats locus within the human complement C2 gene is associated with a retroposon derived from a human endogenous retrovirus. J Exp Med 1992; 175:1783–1787.
83 Yang Z, Yu CY: A comparison of the human and mouse MHC complement gene cluster (MCGC): Gene duplications and sequence conservations (submitted).
84 Kawaguchi H, O'hUigin C, Klein J: Evolution of primate C4 and CYP21 genes; in Klein J, Klein D (eds): Molecular evolution of the major histocompatibility complex. Heidelberg, Springer, 1991, pp 357–381.
85 Schneider PM, Carroll MC, Alper CA, Rittner C, Whitehead AS, Yunis EJ, Colten HR: Polymorphism of human complement C4 and steroid 21-hydroxylase genes. Restriction fragment length polymorphisms revealing structural deletions, homoduplications, and size variants. J Clin Invest 1986;78:650–657.
86 Raum D, Awdeh Z, Anderson J, Strong L, Granados J, Teran L, Giblett E, Yunis EJ, Alper CA: Human C4 haplotypes with duplicated C4A or C4B. Am J Hum Genet 1984;36: 72–79.
87 Chu X, Braun-Heimer L, Rittner C, Schneider PM: Identification of the recombination site within the steroid 21-hydroxylase gene (CYP21) of the HLA-B47, DR7 haplotype. Exp Clin Immunogenet 1992;9:80–85.
88 Donohoue PA, Guethlein L, Collins MM, Dop CV, Migeon CJ, Bias WB, Schmeckpeper BJ: The HLA-A3, Cw6, B47, DR7 extended haplotypes in salt losing 21-hydroxylase deficiency and in the Old Order Amish: Identical class I antigens and class II alleles with at least two crossover sites in the class III region. Tissue Antigens 1995;46:163–172.
89 Yang Z, Mendoza AR, Zipf W, Yu CY: Modular variations of HLA class III genes RP, complement C4, steroid 21-hydroxylase CYP21 and tenascin TNX (RCCX): A mechanism for gene deletions and disease associations. GenBank 1998; Accession number: AF086641.

90 Rupert KL, Rennebohm RM, Yu CY: An unequal crossover between the RCCX modules of the HLA leading to the presence of a *CYP21B* gene and a tenascin *TNXB/TNXA-RP2* recombinant between *C4A* and *C4B* genes in a patient with juvenile rheumatoid arthritis. Exp Clin Immunogenet 1999, in press.
91 Speiser PW, White PC: Structure of the human RD gene: A highly conserved gene in the class III region of the major histocompatibility complex. DNA 1989;745–751.
92 Cheng J, Macon KJ, Volanakis JE: cDNA cloning and characterization of the protein encoded by RD, a gene located in the class III region of the human major histocompatibility complex. Biochem J 1993;294:589–593.
93 Surowy CS, Hoganson G, Gosink J, Stunk K, Spritz RA: The human RD protein is closely related to nuclear RNA-binding proteins and has been highly conserved. Gene 1990;90:299–302.
94 Levi-Strauss M, Carroll MC, Steinmetz M, Meo T: A previously undetected MHC gene with an unusual periodic structure. Science 1988;240:201–204.
95 Qu XD, Yang Z, Zhang S, Shen L, Dangel AW, Hughes JH, Redman KL, Wu LC, Yu CY: The human DEVH- box protein Ski2w is located in nucleoli and ribosomes. Nucleic Acids Res 1998;26:4068–4077.
96 Dangel AW, Shen L, Mendoza AR, Wu L-C, Yu CY: Human helicase gene SKI2W in the HLA class III region exhibits striking structural similarities to the yeast antiviral gene SKI2 and to the human gene KIAA0052: Emergence of a new gene family. Nucleic Acids Res 1995;23:2120–2126.
97 Fuller-Pace FV: RNA helicase: Modulators of RNA structure. Trends Cell Biol 1994;4:271–274.
98 Masison D, Blanc A, Ribas JC, Carroll K, Sonenberg N, Wickner RB: Decoying the cap- mRNA degradation system by a double stranded RNA virus and poly(A)$^-$ mRNA surveillance by a yeast antiviral system. Mol Cell Biol 1995;15:2763–2771.
99 Widner WR, Wickner RB: Evidence that the SKI antiviral system of *Saccharomyces cerevisiae* acts by blocking expression of viral mRNA. Mol Cell Biol 1993;13:4331–4341.
100 Jacobs Anderson J, Parker R: The 3′ to 5′ degradation of yeast mRNAs is a general mechanism for mRNA turnover that requires the SK12 DEVH box protein and 3′ to 5′ exonucleases of the exosome complex. EMBO J 1998;17:1497–1506.
101 Yang Z, Shen L, Dangel AW, Wu LC, Yu CY: Four ubiquitously expressed genes, RD-SKI2W-DOM3Z-RP1, are present between complement component genes factor B and C4 in the class III region of the HLA. Genomics 1998;53:338–347.
102 Paulsen JE, Capowski EE, Strome S: Phenotypic and molecular analysis of *mes*-3, a maternal-effect gene required for proliferation and viability of the germ line in *C. elegans*. Genetics 1995;141:1383–1398.
103 Mauff G, Luther B, Schneider PM, Rittner C, Stradmann-Bellinghausen B, Dawkins R, Moulds JM: Reference typing report for complement component C4. Exp Clin Immunogenet 1998;15:249–260.
104 Geserik G, Otremba P, Schröder H, Stradmann-Bellinghausen B, Schneider PM: Reference typing report for complement factor B. Exp Clin Immunogenet 1998;15:261–263.
105 Lennon G, Auffray C, Polymeropoulos M, Soares MB: An integrated molecular analysis of genomes and their expression. Genomics 1996;33:151–152.

Experimental and Clinical Immunogenetics

Exp Clin Immunogenet 1998;15:231–234

Received: May 23, 1998
Revised version: July 9, 1998

Marina Botto

Rheumatology Section, Division of Medicine, Imperial College School of Medicine, London, UK

C1q Knock-Out Mice for the Study of Complement Deficiency in Autoimmune Disease

Key Words
Complement
Deficiency
Autoimmunity
Gene targeting
Mice

Abstract
In humans, homozygous deficiency of the first component of the classical pathway of complement, C1q, is a powerful disease susceptibility factor for the development of systemic lupus erythematosus (SLE). This strong association indicates that a functional activity of C1q protects from the development of SLE. Studies in vitro have shown that C1q can bind apoptotic keratinocytes suggesting that it may have an important role in the clearance of apoptotic cells. C1q-deficient mice, generated by gene targeting, showed an increased mortality and 25% of the mice had histological evidence of glomerulonephritis characterised by multiple apoptotic cell bodies and immune deposits, assessed by immunofluorescence and electron microscopy. These observations are compatible with the hypothesis that C1q deficiency causes autoimmunity by an impaired clearance of apoptotic cells.

Complement Deficiency and Lupus

Hereditary deficiency of proteins of the classical pathway of the complement system is strongly associated with the development of systemic lupus erythematosus (SLE). There is a hierarchy of both prevalence and severity of disease according to the position of the deficient protein in the classical pathway. Homozygous deficiency of C1q is associated with a greater than 90% prevalence of severe disease, whereas C2 deficiency is associated with SLE of moderate severity in approximately 33% of subjects, and C3 deficiency is only rarely associated with SLE. These clinical observations lead to the hypothesis that there is a physiological activity of the early part of the classical pathway of complement that protects against the development of SLE [1, 2].

In humans, homozygous deficiency of the first component of the complement system, C1q, is the most powerful susceptibility genet-

KARGER

Fax +41 61 306 12 34
E-Mail karger@karger.ch
www.karger.com

0254–9670/98/0154–0231$17.50/0

Accessible online at:
http://BioMedNet.com/karger

Marina Botto
Rheumatology Section, Division of Medicine
Imperial College School of Medicine, Hammersmith Campus
Du Cane Road, London W12 0NN (UK)
Tel. +44 181 383 2316, Fax +44 181 743 3109

ic factor for the development of systemic lupus erythematosus (SLE). The vast majority of patients with C1q deficiency develop a syndrome closely related to SLE [3]. The disease is typically of early onset and is often very severe. It has been described equally in males and females and rash, typically of a photosensitive nature, has been reported as a prominent feature in 36 out of the 41 patients described in the literature.

Although the phenotype of disease varies between patients, the fact that C1q deficiency is sufficient to cause SLE in almost all humans, identifies a pivotal role for this molecule. The challenge is to identify the relevant physiological activity that can explain this strong association. Here we will discuss two candidate activities that have been implicated: one is the role of the classical pathway in the processing of immune complexes (ICs) and the other is the possible role of C1q in the clearance of apoptotic cells. This is a newly described function that has recently been suggested by studies in vitro and in vivo.

Complement and the Processing of IC

In support of the hypothesis that the role of the complement in the processing of IC plays a key role in the protection against the development of SLE there are several studies showing that IC are cleared with a very abnormal pattern in the presence of either acquired or hereditary hypocomplementaemia [4–7]. The classical pathway of complement inhibits the formation of large IC lattices and promotes the uptake by the mononuclear phagocytic system. The most striking abnormalities of IC processing in complement-deficient patients is the impaired uptake of ICs in the mononuclear phagocytic system of the liver and the complete absence of uptake into the spleen [8].

Defective processing of IC could result in large ICs escaping the mononuclear phagocytic system and depositing in tissues where they can trigger an inflammatory response with the release of autoantigens leading to the development of an autoantibody response.

Mechanisms of Clearance of Apoptotic Cells – A Role for C1q

In support of the second hypothesis there are some recent observations in vitro and in vivo indicating that C1q may be implicated in the clearance of apoptotic cells. Apoptosis, or programmed cell death, is a physiological mechanism for eliminating damaged or unwanted cells without initiating an inflammatory response. Apoptotic cells or the resulting cellular fragments, apoptotic bodies, are subjected to a rapid receptor-mediated ingestion by macrophages or resident tissue phagocytes. One of the earliest features of apoptosis is prominent surface blebbing. These small blebs arise from the fragmented rough endoplasmic reticulum and are highly enriched in lupus autoantigens such as Ro and La [9–11]. In addition to the enrichment of lupus autoantigens within apoptotic surface blebs, as part of the process of apoptosis, there is active translocation of anionic phospholipids, particularly phosphatidylserine, from the inner to the outer lamella of the bilayer of the cell membrane [12]. From these data, the hypothesis has developed that apoptotic cells may be the major source of highly concentrated autoantigens driving the autoimmune response in SLE.

Korb and Ahearn [13] have recently demonstrated that when human keratinocytes become apoptotic they develop the capacity to directly bind to C1q in the absence of antibodies, suggesting that C1q may play a role in the recognition of apoptotic bodies. A hypothesis that follows from all of these observations is that, in situations where the removal of apoptotic cells is abnormal, as might occur in C1q deficiency, ineffectively cleared apoptotic cells may become the source of autoantigens that can stimulate the immune response. This hypothesis is supported by the results of our recent studies in complement-deficient mice. In order to work on the problem of how complement deficiency causes the development of SLE, we developed strains of mice with C1q deficiency by gene targeting. Our observations in these mice suggest that C1q may play a role in the physiological clearance mechanisms of apoptotic cells and thereby offer a potential explanation for the association of C1q deficiency with SLE.

Complement Deficiency and the Clearance of Apoptotic Cells

The coding region of the first exon of the *C1qa* gene [14] was disrupted by homologous recombination, generating C1q-deficient mice. Animals were fully viable and fertile. Amongst the C1q-deficient mice of a mixed genetic background (129/Ola × C57BL/6), high titres of antinuclear antibodies were detected in approximately 54% compared with 33% of strain-matched controls. Approximately 25% of the C1q-deficient mice, aged 8 months, developed severe crescentic glomerulonephritis, characterised by the presence of immune deposits and multiple apoptotic cell bodies in injured glomeruli [15]. Amongst mice without glomerulonephritis there were significantly greater numbers of glomerular apoptotic bodies in the C1q-deficient mice compared with control animals. These striking histological features, not reported in humans with C1q deficiency, coupled with the usually short clearance time of apoptotic cells in injured glomeruli [16], suggest that impaired clearance of apoptotic cells is likely to be a primary defect in C1q-deficient mice. The hypothesis that there may be a defect in the clearance of apoptotic cells in C1q-deficient mice is consistent with the findings of Korb and Ahearn [13] showing that C1q binds to apoptotic keratinocytes in an antibody-independent pattern. Amongst the C1q-deficient mice, the presence of autoantibodies did not correlate with either the presence or the severity of the renal involvement. We therefore hypothesize that C1q may bind to the surface of apoptotic cells promoting their physiological clearance without the development of inflammation. In situations where the removal of apoptotic cells is abnormal, as might occur in C1q deficiency, these cells may provide a major source of autoantigens that drive the autoimmune response in SLE and related diseases.

Dysregulation of apoptotic cell processing is emerging as a new hypothesis to explain important features in the development of autoimmune disease associated with C1q deficiency. An inappropriately high rate of apoptosis or a defect in the clearance of apoptotic cells may promote the accumulation of abnormal cells that might drive an autoimmune response. Although only a minority of patients with SLE have inherited homozygous complement deficiency, a majority have acquired complement deficiency as part of the disease process. The hypothesis that complement deficiency causes defects in the mechanisms of processing of apoptotic cells is therefore relevant to the majority of patients with SLE and could have future therapeutic implications.

Acknowledgment

This work was supported by Arthritis Research Campaign.

References

1 Walport MJ, Morgan BP: Complement deficiency and disease. Immunol Today 1991;12:301–306.

2 Lachmann PJ, Walport MJ: Deficiency of the effector mechanisms of the immune response and autoimmunity; in Whelan J (ed): Ciba Foundation Symposium: Autoimmunity and Autoimmune Diseases. Wiley, Chichester, 1987, vol 129, pp 149–171.

3 Bowness P, Davies KA, Norsworthy PJ, Athanassiou P, Taylor Wiedeman J, Borysiewicz LK, Meyer PA, Walport MJ: Hereditary C1q deficiency and systemic lupus erythematosus. Q J Med 1994;87:455–464.

4 Davies KA, Schifferli JA, Walport MJ: Complement deficiency and immune complex disease. Springer Semin Immunopathol 1994;15: 397–416.

5 Lobatto S, Daha MR, Breedveld FC, Pauwels EK, Evers Schouten JH, Voetman A, Cats A, Van Es LA: Abnormal clearance of soluble aggregates of human immunoglobulin G in patients with systemic lupus erythematosus. Clin Exp Immunol 1988;72:55–59.

6 Davies KA, Peters AM, Beynon HLC, Walport MJ: Immune complex processing in patients with systemic lupus erythematosus: In vivo imaging and clearance studies. J Clin Invest 1992;90:2075–2083.

7 Halma C, Daha MR, Camps JAJ, Evers-Schouten JH, Pauwel EKJ, van Es LA: Deficiency of complement C3 is associated with accelerated removal of soluble ^{123}I-labelled aggregates of IgG from the circulation. Clin Exp Immunol 1992;90: 394–400.

8 Davies KA, Peters AM, Beynon HLC, Erlendsson K, Steinsson K, Valdimarsson H, Walport MJ: Splenic uptake of immune complexes in man is complement-dependent. J Immunol 1993;151: 3866–3873.

9 Casciola-Rosen LA, Anhalt G, Rosen A: Autoantigens targeted in systemic lupus erythematosus are clustered in tow populations of surface structures on apoptotic keratinocytes. J Exp Med 1994;179:1317–1330.

10 Rosen A, Casciola-Rosen LA, Ahearn J: Novel packages of viral and self-antigens are generated during apoptosis. J Exp Med 1995;181: 1557–1561.

11 Casciola-Rosen LA, Rosen A, Petri M, Schlissel M: Surface blebs on apoptotic cells are sites of enhanced procoagulant activity: Implications for coagulation events and antigenic spread in systemic lupus erythematosus. Proc Natl Acad Sci USA 1996;93:1624–1629.

12 Fadok VA, Voelker DR, Campbell PA, Cohen JJ, Bratton DL, Henson PM: Exposure of phosphatidylserine on the surface of apoptotic lymphocytes triggers specific recognition and removal by macrophages. J Immunol 1992;148:2207–2216.

13 Korb LC, Ahearn JM: C1q binds directly and specifically to surface blebs of apoptotic human keratinocytes. Complement deficiency and systemic lupus erythematosus revisited. J Immunol 1997;158:4525–4528.

14 Petry F, McClive PJ, Botto M, Morley BJ, Morahan G, Loos M: The mouse C1q genes are clustered on chromosome 4 and show conservation of gene organisation. Immunogenetics 1996;43:370–376.

15 Botto M, Dell'Agnola C, Bygrave AE, Thompson M, Cook HT, Petry F, Loos M, Pandolfi PP, Walport MJ: Homozygous C1q deficiency causes glomerulonephritis associated with multiple apoptotic bodies. Nat Genet 1998;19:56–59.

16 Baker AJ, Mooney A, Hughes J, Lombardi D, Johnson RJ, Savill J: Mesangial cell apoptosis: The major mechanism for resolution of glomerular hypercellularity in experimental mesangial proliferative nephritis. J Clin Invest 1994;94:2105–2116.

Experimental and Clinical Immunogenetics

Exp Clin Immunogenet 1998;15:235–243

Received: May 23, 1998
Revised version: July 2, 1998

M.J. Hobart

Department of Biological Sciences,
De Montfort University,
Leicester, UK

Evolution of the Terminal Complement Genes: Ancient and Modern

Key Words
Evolution
Complement
C6
C7
C8
C9

Abstract
The data on the structure and relationships of the TCC genes are reviewed and a model is presented for the processes of gene duplication by which the modern genes might have evolved. Data on variations of the overall gene numbers and relationships in modern species are also reviewed, together with the polymorphisms found in man. The apparent contradictions of lack of allelic association between markers and lack of direct evidence for recombination in the C6/C7 gene region is also discussed.

Although what follows is based upon established data, the data are incomplete and leave significant enigmas. Consequently, there is a large measure of speculation in the conclusions which are reached and a good probability that they will prove erroneous. However, new data do not seem likely to become available in the near future, so perhaps it is time to be provocative.

The data for the topic of ancient evolution come very largely from studies of the structure and relationships of the human terminal complement genes C6, C7, C8A C8B and C9. They are supplanted by studies on the C9 of two teleost fishes: trout [1] and the Japanese puffer fish (*Fugu rubripes*). The close relationships of the terminal complement components has been proven since the cloning and analysis of the cDNAs for the five components [2–8] and these studies left no doubt that they have arisen from a common ancestor by a process of gene duplication. They also showed that the terminal complement components are apparently fairly typical mosaic proteins, composed at least in part of modules (domains) which are recognised in other proteins.

The first gene structure to be investigated was C9 [9], a study which revealed a number of interesting features, notably that the pro-

KARGER
Fax + 41 61 306 12 34
E-Mail karger@karger.ch
www.karger.com

0254–9670/98/0154–0235$17.50/0

Accessible online at:
http://BioMedNet.com/karger

M.J. Hobart
Department of Biological Sciences
De Montfort University, Leicester LE1 9BH (UK)
Tel. +44 116 255 1551, ext. 8111, Fax +44 116 257 7135
E-Mail mhobart@dmu.ac.uk

tein modules do not (in most cases) correspond to the exons. This is an unusual, though not unique, pattern. Studies on the structure of the C6, C7 and the two C8 genes progressed in parallel in three laboratories [10–13]. Although the large C6 and C7 genes presented a greater task than the C8 genes, they also provided much more critical data because of their complexity and it became clear that the gene architectures were startlingly similar. The term 'architecture' is used here to describe the positions and, most especially, the phase types of the introns which were all identical in C6 and C7 and most were the same as in C9 (where relevant). It has now been shown that they are, in fact, the same in all five genes [14] and that this feature is shared by *Fugu* C9 [15].

The genes are in two clusters in humans, C6 near C7 but removed from C9 on chromosome 5 [16–21] and C8A and C8B on chromosome 1 [22, 23]. Both C6/C7 and C8A/C8B are arranged in 3′-to-3′orientation [21, 24, 25]. The position and orientation of C9 relative to C6/C7 is not known, but it is at least 2.5 mbp distant [21].

Ancient Evolution

Because the intron phase types are both identical in all members of the gene family and jumbled with respect to type along the genes, it must be the case that the duplications of the genes happened after these characteristics were established. The events prior to the duplications can only be guessed at: almost certainly a conventional assembly of the proto-gene by exon shuffling to bring together the exons encoding the protein modules, followed by a surprising elimination of the primitive introns and replacement by the 'modern' ones. These processes may have been simultaneous or either may have happened first. However, this is truly ancient history, as sharks have a fully functional complement system [26] and there is little doubt that the gene duplication events happened before humans and sharks shared an ancestor (about 400,000,000 years ago).

The principal questions on which we can speculate are: what was the proto-gene like and in what order did the gene duplication events happen? In addressing this, it would be attractive to present a suggested history in which the components could be imagined as having function at an early stage and which can progress to something like the modern system very rapidly (i.e. with very few steps). Some evolutionary steps have a higher 'tariff' than others: inversion duplications are relatively unusual compared with tandem duplication by unequal crossover; polyploid duplication (chromosome duplication) probably last happened in our ancestry before chromosomal sex determination (fish); but deletion of genes or parts of genes is common (including being a cause of some human gene defects).

I would argue (strongly for at least C7) that the proto-gene was more like C6 than any of the other modern genes. The basis for the argument is that it is very difficult to build up a gene when the introns are in the 'wrong' places and of 'random' types (fig. 1). The 5′ ends of the C6 and C7 genes are the clearest evidence of this point: the only realistic model for their evolution is that they derive from an ancestor which encoded two N-terminal thrombospondin modules prior to the shifting of the introns and from a later ancestor in which the intron shift had happened. C7 could only have evolved by deletion from this ancestor because C6 could not evolve by accretion as its N-terminal thrombospondin domain is encoded in part by two exons (fig. 2). The similar argument for the evolution of the other genes is weaker and relies more heavily on the notion that deletion is a relatively easy

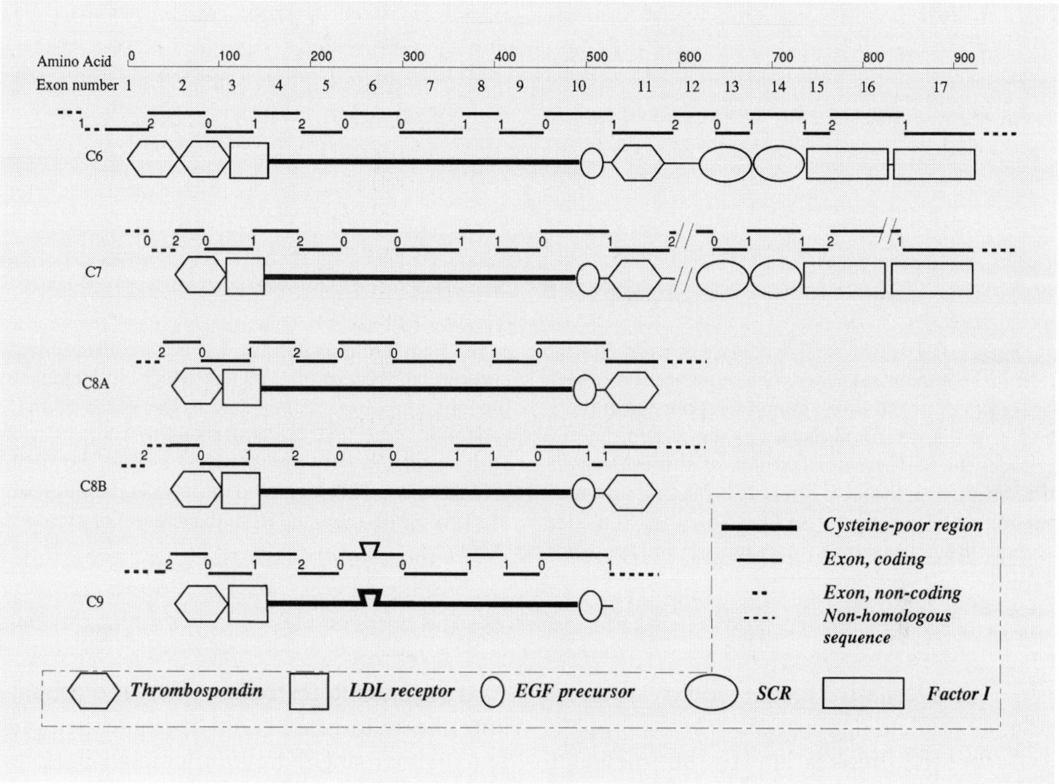

Fig. 1. The exons of the terminal complements components. The exons are depicted as staggered black bars. The large numbers above the bars are the exon numbers starting from the first protein-coding exon, and the small numbers between the ends of the bars show the phase of the corresponding intron. The homology of both exon length and phase is very strong between C6, C7, C8A, C8B and C9, but lengths are not precisely represented in this diagram. Note that (with the exception of exon 14) the exons do not correspond to the protein homology units. Figure and legend are revised from J Immunol 1995;154:5188–5194.

step, whereas adding a further set of modules very imperfectly mapped to the exons at the 3′ end of the C6 and C7 genes would be a considerable feat of gene manipulation.

A challenge to strictly rational argument is to construct a history for the gene duplication processes which is reasonably parsimonious, especially as concerns events which seem to happen rarely in evolution. The model which I wish to suggest is shown schematically in figure 3. The first event is a tandem duplication of the proto-gene. Following this, the ancestor of the small (C8 and C9) genes diverges by deletion from the ancestor of the large (C6 and C7) genes. In order for the final arrangement of the C6, C7 and C9 genes to be fitted into the proposed history, the gene in question must be the 5′ member of the pair. This means that the deletions from its 3′ end would have happened at the end closest to the other

Exon 2

	C6 Thrombospondin 1 (C-terminus)	C6 Thrombospondin 2 (N-terminus) Others Thrombospondin 1
C6	gQIVVDKYYQENFCEQICSKQETRECNWQRCP	INCLLGDFGPWSDCDPCIEKQ
C7	rASSP	VNCQWDFYAPWSECNGCTKTQ
C8A	nRVRRAATPAA	VTCQLSNWSEWTDCFPCQDKK
C8B	gGERPHSFGSNAVNKSFAKSRQMRSVDVTLMP	IDCELSSWSSWTTCDPCQKKR
C9	rYDPELTESSGSASH	IDCRMSPWSEWSQCDPCLRQM

Fig. 2. The amino acid sequences of exon 2 of the terminal complement genes. The sequences have been broken to show the strong homologies present at the 3′ end, and the weak homologies at the 5′ end. Exon 2 encodes the 5′ (N-terminal) region of a thrombospondin repeat in all the TCC genes. It is the first thrombospondin in all the genes other than C6, in which it is the second. In C6, the exon encodes at its 5′ end the 3′ end of the first thrombospondin, but in the other genes it encodes an N-terminal region which is lacking in obvious homology, either among the genes or more generally. Note that the length of this coding region varies markedly between the genes, as does the amino acid sequence. It is suggested that this is the end result of a process of 'nibbling' from the end of the genes.

gene. An alternative model would be for the original tandem duplication to be incomplete and for the duplication to be mediated through the homologous thrombospondin domain sequences which form both the 5′ components of all the terminal complement genes and also the 3′ component of C8-like genes. Next, a major inversion duplication takes place involving both genes, leaving the pairs 3′-to-3′. The last duplication is the polyploid duplication which separates the C8 gene ancestors from the others. All subsequent events are deletions: of the large genes in the case of the C8 ancestors, probably bringing the small genes close together, and of one of the small genes in the case of the other cluster. The model satisfies the parsimony criteria quite well, as any mechanism must include at least one event each of the processes of inversion, tandem and polyploid duplication and one major deletion or insertion. The model additionally requires only two deletions, both of them major.

It is possible to imagine that the original long and short genes could have encoded proteins which might have interacted in some useful way. The inversion and polyploid duplications would have multiplied the genes without upsetting gene dosage and might well have happened in a brief time-span, leaving the raw material for fine-tuning by selected deletions.

The model also makes two testable predictions: the strong prediction that C9 will prove to be oriented in the same sense as its nearest neighbour of the C6/C7 pair and the weak prediction that that neighbour will be C6. It is also suggested that the deletion of the 'spare' gene (if it was deleted and not merely modified and currently undiscovered) might have coincided with the 'trimming' of the 5′ region of the C7 gene. This is a weak prediction and the model would not totally fall if C9 were found closest to C7.

The detailed changes which differentiate the individual genes are both relatively small compared with the very large-scale events

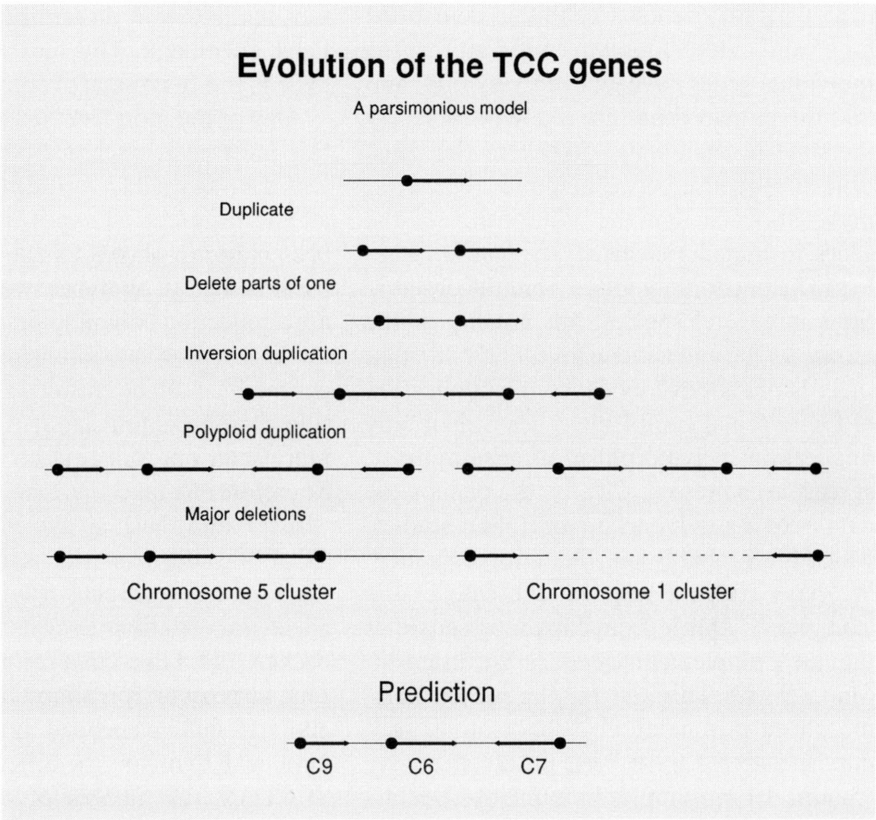

Fig. 3. A model for the duplications of the TCC genes. The figure shows a parsimonious model for the duplications and other events which might have led to the arrangement of the terminal complement genes as they are found in man. The 5′ ends of the genes are indicated by a knob ('head') and the 3′ ends by an arrowhead ('tail'). Note that it is essential for the deletion of the 3′ end of the ancestor of the C8 and C9 genes to have occurred on the 5′ member of the original duplicated pair.

postulated above. Further understanding of them probably requires a better knowledge of the structure/function relationships. This may come from both protein studies (both full function and yeast two-hybrid interaction) and from comparative studies of the genes in both mammals and other vertebrates. It would, of course, be wonderful to identify and analyse the terminal complement genes or their precursors in lower vertebrates (e.g. cyclostomes or chordates). Results from such studies could reveal the truth about the speculations with which we currently attempt to satisfy ourselves.

Intermediate Evolution

Having emphasised the interest in working out the duplication processes for terminal complement genes, let me now suggest that the stability which I have assumed from fish to humans may be less true than is demanded for a valid model. I remain confident that the individual genes have evolved very little and that the human genes are likely to represent the state in mammals, subject to the usual drift of sequence between species. However, my confidence that the relationship of the genes in humans is strictly typical is rather less. The uncertainty arises from the observations in several species, but notably in the mouse for C6 and the dog for C7 [27, 28], that there is phenotypic evidence for duplication of the terminal complement genes. Not only duplication: polymorphism of gene number, at least as expressed. Clearly, the phenotypic data require the backup of DNA studies, which are probably not likely to be funded. We have still not resolved the case of the 'complex' C7 allele from Japan, presented at the last Complement Genetics Workshop in Mainz (1989). This, too, may be due to a polymorphism in gene number, and similar phenotype patterns have been observed among Chinese serum samples [unpubl. obs.]. However, if there is instability of gene number, then there may be opportunities for instability in gene relationships and the finding that the pairs are 3′-to-3′ may be an accident, or, less plausibly, due to a familial tendency to undergo inversion.

Modern Evolution: Polymorphisms and Defects of the C6 and C7 Genes in Humans

The terminal complement genes have long attracted attention by their polymorphisms: much less extreme than those of C4, but quite diverse and in several cases, especially in C6 and C7, present at high allele frequencies. The first hint of this diversity was observed in C6 by Chester Alper, using his recently developed agarose gel electrophoresis and immunofixation method with an antiserum provided by Peter Lachmann. This hint was consolidated by IEF and functional overlay studies [29].

One of the more detailed issues covered at this meeting is reference typing of markers. One day, we shall know the molecular bases of all the different allotypes. However, as has been elegantly shown for the C4 markers, the truth is that all allotypes (well most, at least) are a reflection of haplotypes of differences in the DNA. The maximum number of differences which can be encoded at a single nucleotide position is four, an it is unusual to find more than one substitution within a codon. Therefore, to take the cases of C6 and C7, which I know best, all alleles of C6 are either 'A' or 'B' at the exon 3 locus which is responsible for that venerable polymorphism. Rare alleles are variations elsewhere on an 'A' or 'B' background. Given that recombination in the gene does occur, it is almost certain that some allotypes will be encoded by different combinations of their specific difference with 'A' or 'B'. Thus, the number of molecular differences may be appreciably smaller than we currently believe. Few new polymorphisms have revealed themselves during the investigation of C6 deficiencies and one which did was intronic and thoroughly peculiar, involving a combined insertion and deletion.

To immediately contradict this statement, there are more C7 variants than we first thought, based on phenotypic data. In Caucasians, charge variants of C7 are infrequent (about 0.01 allele frequency). However, there are three known expressed polymorphisms (S367T; T565P, M/N; and T576S), only one of which is phenotypically detectable and this only by the subtleness of a monoclonal antibody. They have second allele frequencies in the range 0.1–0.4 (in North Europeans).

Although the phenotypic methods still have their place, they are rapidly being replaced by DNA-based methods, which also offer a considerable number of other markers. The great advantage of DNA methods for marker studies in deficiency is that it is possible to type the defective genes (though one referee criticised a paper on the grounds that we should be protein typing a deficient individual!) and even predict what protein they would make and subsequently find it [30] (so the referee was only mostly wrong). Furthermore, DNA markers and especially the collected markers which comprise haplotypes were quickly recognised as having great potential for diagnosis, even before gene structures were known [31, 32].

More recent work, much related to the investigation of molecular defects, has led to the discovery of a number of single base substitution polymorphisms. We have used up to 11 of these, all present at allele frequencies above 0.1, defining some 2,056 potential haplotypes, in the study of both defects and of diversity in human populations. In view of the comparatively modest number of individuals and, above all, families tested, a surprising number of different haplotypes have been observed. It is difficult to count these: unless investigating extensive or three-generation families, heterozygosity at more than one locus can make the assignment of halopytes impossible. Thus, the greater the number of loci investigated, the fewer individuals can be unequivocally analysed. However, it is certain that several tens of haplotypes are present in the population. This diversity is something of a surprise, since the gene region under consideration spans only about 320 kbp and, to the best of my knowledge, no meiosis involving a new recombination within or between the C6 and C7 genes has been observed in either humans or animals. Nevertheless, there is, in most cases, a startling lack of allelic association between the markers.

In contrast, associations between marker haplotypes and specific disease alleles are generally very strong. In fact, we have observed only 5 cases where there are recombinant haplotypes associated with defects. Two are in populations where a single cause of C7 deficiency predominates: exon 7 and 8 deletion among the Irish [33, 34] and a missense mutation in exon 9 which predominates among Moroccan Jews [33, 35, 36]. In both cases, the recombinations are between the most distal C6 marker and the rest of the haplotype. The other 3 are in C6-deficient South Africans, among whom 1 defect is about 5 times more common than the other 2 so far discovered [35, 36]. The common defect is a deletion of 1 of the 7 G nucleotides from cDNA 879, exon 6 [37], 90% associated with single haplotype. The other two haplotypes differ at the distal end of the C7 gene (2 cases) and both the proximal (3′) and the distal end (1 case). The other 2 defects in South Africa are probably 'African', as they were first reported in African Americans [38, 39] and we have also found them in a British subject of African extraction. There are two haplotypes associated with the more common of these alleles, differing at a proximal C7 locus. However, the two proximal C7 loci in question are *Taq*I sites, with the less common allele having the site absent. This is quite probably due to mutation of the central CpG dinucleotide.

Another deficiency association which seems quite strong is that of the subtotal deficiencies of C6 and C7 [30, 40]. Homozygotes for this condition are distinctly rare and 2 have been reported in the UK. The defective chromosome has a characteristic haplotype and heterozygotes with the molecular defects and haplotype have been found from Russia, through Germany to South Africa. However, in addition, recombinants have been found in whom only a single defect and its associated 'half haplotype' are found. This seems likely to have arisen by recombinational splitting rather than joining.

Thus, there is therefore strong evidence both in favour of recombination within and between the C6 and C7 genes and in favour of considerable stability of the region, at least comparable with the life span of a molecular defect. These themselves include chromosomes which have certainly survived long enough to spread across Europe and Africa, before being transplanted to new continents since the advent of commercial intercontinental navigation. There is no evidence that the C6 and C7 genes have a recombination 'hot spot', rather that the recombination is fairly uniform along the region, though perhaps less at the 5′ end of C7.

What now follows is something of a list of unanswered questions. Why are the C6 A/B and *Msp*I alleles in such strong association among North Europeans, while among other groups, apparently no further away than the Picos de Europa mountain range in Spain, the association does not exist? Why are there stronger allelic associations between alleles at loci further apart than those which are closer?

Finally

Why is it that many of the multitude of markers are common to all human population groups, in many cases at similar or very similar gene frequencies? Do these polymorphisms date from our pre-human ancestors and, if so, how did they pass through a speciation bottleneck? If they are specifically human, was there a period during early human evolution when our genes were particularly mutable? The terminal complement genes connect us to our ancient past in a rather special way. They also remind us that we are closely connected to each other.

References

1 Tomlinson S, Stanley KK, Esser AF: Domain structure, functional activity, and polymerization of trout complement protein-C9. Dev Comp Immunol 1993;17:67–76.

2 Stanley KK, Kocher H-P, Luzio JP, Jackson P, Tschopp J: The sequence and topology of human complement component C9. EMBO 1985;4:375–382.

3 Haefliger J-A, Tschopp J, Nardelli D, Wahli W, Kocher H-P, Tosi M, Stanley KK: Complementary DNA cloning of C8beta and its sequence homology to C9. Biochemistry. 1987;26:3551–3556.

4 Howard OM, Rao AG, Sodetz JM: Complementary DNA and derived amino acid sequence of the beta subunit of human complement component C8: Identification of a close structural and ancestral relationship to the alpha subunit and C9. Biochemistry 1987;26:3565–3570.

5 Rao AG, Howard OMZ, Ng SC, Whitehead AS, Colten HR, Sodetz JM: Complementary DNA and derived amino acid sequence for the alpha subunit of human complement component C8: Evidence for the existence of a separate alpha subunit messenger RNA. Biochemistry 1987;26:3556–3564.

6 Haefliger J-A, Tschopp J, Vial N, Jenne DE: Complete primary structure and functional characterisation of the sixth component of the human complement system. J Biol Chem 1989;264:18041–18051.

7 DiScipio RG, Hugli TE: The molecular architecture of human complement component C6. J Biol Chem 1989;264i:16197–16206.

8 DiScipio RG, Chakravarti DN, Muller-Eberhard HJ, Fey GH: The structure of human complement component C7 and the C5b-7 complex. J Biol Chem 1988;263:549–560.

9 Marazziti D, Eggertsen G, Fey GH, Stanley KK: Relationships between gene and protein structure in human complement component C9. Biochemistry 1988;27:6529–6534.

10 Hobart MJ, Fernie B, DiScipio RG: Structure of the human C6 gene. Biochemistry 1993;32:6198–6205.

11 Kaufmann T, Rittner C, Schneider PM: The human complement component C8 gene: Structure and phylogenetic relationship. Hum Genet 1993;92:69–75.

12 Michelotti GA, Snider JV, Sodetz JM: Genomic organization of human complement protein C8α and further examination of its linkage to C8β. Hum Genet 1995;95:513–518.

13 Hobart MJ, Fernie B, DiScipio RG: Structure of the Human C7 gene and comparison with the C7, C8A, C8B and C9 genes. J Immunol 1995;154:5188–5194.

14 Witzel-Schlömp K, Späth PJ, Hobart MJ, Fernie B, Rittner C, Kaufmann T, Schneider PM: The human complement C9 gene: Identification of two mutations causing deficiency and revision of the gene structure. J Immunol 1997;158:5043–5049.
15 Yeo GSH, Elgar G, Sandford R, Brenner S: Cloning and sequencing of complement component C9(1) and its linkage to DOC-2 in the pufferfish *Fugu rubripes*. Gene 1997; 200:203–211.
16 Abbott C, West L, Povey S, Jeremiah S, Murad Z, DiScipio R, Frey G: The gene for human complement component C9 mapped to chromosome 5 by polymerase chain reaction. Genomics 1989;4:606–609.
17 Rogde S, Myklebost O, Stanley K, van Kessel G: The gene for human complement component C9 is on chromosome 5. Genomics 1989;5: 149–152.
18 Jeremiah SJ, Abbott CM, Murad Z, Povey S, Thomas HJ, Solomon E, DiScipio R, Fey GH: The assignment of the genes coding human complement components C6 and C7 to chromosome 5. Ann Hum Genet 1990;54:141–147.
19 Rogde S, Myklebost O, Olving JH, Kyrkjebø HT, Jonassen R, Olaisen B, Gedde-Dahl T: The human genes for complement components 6 (C6) and 9 (C9) are closely linked on chromosome 5. J Med Genet 1991; 28:587–590.
20 Coto E, Martinez-Navez E, Dominguez O, DiScipio R, Urra JM, Lopez-Larrea C: DNA polymorphisms and linkage relationship of the human complement component C6, C7 and C9 genes. Immunogenetics 1991;33:184–187.
21 Setién F, Alvarez V, Coto E, DiScipio RG, López-Larrea C: A physical map of the human complement component C6, C7 and C9 genes. Immunogenetics 1993;38:341–344.
22 Theriault A, Boyd E, Whaley K, Sodetz JM, Connor JM: Regional chromosome assignment of genes encoding the alpha-subunit and beta-subunit of human complement protein-C8 to 1p32. Hum Genet 1992;88:703–704.
23 Rogde S, Gedde-Dahl T Jr, Teisberg P, Jonassen R, Hoyheim B, Olaisen B: Linkage and association studies with C8A and C8B RFLPs on chromosome 1. Ann Hum Genet 1992; 56:233–242.
24 Hobart MJ, Fernie BA, DiScipio RG, Lachmann PJ: A physical map of the C6 and C7 complement component gene region on chromosome 5p13. Hum Mol Genet 1993;2: 1035–1036.
25 Platteborze PL, Hobart MJ, Sodetz JM: Physical linkage and orientation of the human complement component C8A and C8B genes on chromosome 1p32. Hum Genet 1996; 98:443–446.
26 Jensen JA, Festa E, Smith DS, Cayer M: The complement system of the nurse shark: Haemolytic and comparative characteristics. Science 1981;214:566–569.
27 Eldridge PR, Hobart MJ, Lachmann PJ: The genetics of the sixth and seventh components of complement in the dog: Polymorphism, linkage, locus duplication, and silent alleles. Biochem Genet 1983;21:81–91.
28 Orren A, Wallace ME, Hobart MJ, Lachmann PJ: C6 polymorphism and C6 deficiency in site strains of the mutation-prone Peru-Coppock mice. Complement Inflamm 1989; 6:295–296.
29 Hobart MJ, Lachmann PJ, Alper CA: Polymorphism of human C6; Peeters (ed): Protides of the Biological Fluids. 22nd Colloquium. London, Pergamon Press, 1975, pp 575–580.
30 Fernie BA, Würzner R, Orren A, Morgan BP, Potter PC, Platonov AE, Vershinina IV, Shipulin GA, Lachmann PL, Hobart MJ: Molecular bases of combined subtotal deficiencies of C6 and C7 and their effects in combination with other deficiencies. J Immunol 1996;157: 3648–3657.
31 Coto E, Martinez-Naves E, Dominguez O, Lopez-Larrea C: DNA polymorphism of the human complement component C7 gene in familial deficiencies. Hum Genet 1990;85: 251–252.
32 Potter PC, Warburton C, Würzner R, Orren A, DiScipio R: Association of a 12.5-kilobase allele of the *Msp*I restriction fragment length polymorphism of the C6 gene in patients with total deficiency of the sixth component complement. Exp Clin Immunogenet 1993;10:38–44.
33 Fernie BA, Orren A, Sheehan G, Schlesinger M, Hobart MJ: Molecular bases of C7 deficiency: Three different defects. J Immunol 1997;159: 1019–1026.
34 O'Hara AM, Moran AP, Fernie BA, Connaughton JJ, Orren A, Hobart MJ: Molecular bases of deficiency of the seventh complement component, deletions of exons 7 and 8. Irish J Med Sci (abstract), in press
25 Schlesinger M, Nave Z, Levy Y, Slater PE, Fishelson Z: Prevalence of hereditary properdin, C7 and C8 deficiencies in patients with meningococcal infections. Clin Exp Immunol 1990;81:423.
36 Molad Y, Zimran A, Sidi Y, Pinkhas J: Posttraumatic meningococcemia in a patient with deficiency of the C7 complement component. Isr J Med Sci 1990;26:90–92.
37 Hobart MJ, Fernie BA, Fijen CAP, Orren A: The molecular bases of C6 deficiency in the Western Cape, South Africa (abstract 10M). Abstr 7th Complement Genetics Workshop and Conference, 1998.
38 Nishizaka H, Horiuchi T, Zhu Z-B, Fukumori Y, Nagasawa K, Hayashi K, Krumdieck R, Cobbs CG, Higuchi M, Yasunaga S, Niho Y, Volanakis JE: Molecular bases of inherited human complement component C6 deficiency in two unrelated individuals. J Immunol 1996;156:2309–2315.
39 Zhu ZB, Totemchokchyakarn K, Atkinson TP, Volanakis JE: Molecular defects leading to human complement component C6 deficiency in an African-American family. Clin Exp Immunol 1998;111:91–96.
40 Lachmann PJ, Hobart MJ, Woo P: Combined genetic deficiency of C6 and C7 in man. Clin Exp Immunol 1978;33:193.

Experimental and Clinical Immunogenetics

Exp Clin Immunogenet 1998;15:244–248

Received: May 23, 1998
Revised version: July 14, 1998

Yasuo Fukumori[a]
Takahiko Horiuchi[b]

[a] Osaka Red Cross Blood Center, Osaka, and
[b] 1st Department of Internal Medicine, Kyushu University, Fukuoka, Japan

Terminal Complement Component Deficiencies in Japan

Key Words
Complement deficiency
Genetic analysis
Japan

Abstract
From the serological screening for complement component deficiencies, we found 2 subjects with inherited C5 deficiency (C5D), 4 with C6D, 6 with C7D, 4 with C81 (α-γ subunit) D and 138 with C9D among 145,640 healthy Japanese blood donors. Recently, the genetic bases of some of the C6D, C7D, C81D and C9D Japanese individuals were elucidated using an exon-specific PCR-SSCP method followed by direct sequencing of the target exons.

Introduction

The terminal complement components, C5–C9, are the 5 constituents of the membrane attack complex which work at the final process of the complement system and are assembled on the membrane of target cells. All these proteins are homologous with each other and have a mosaic structure consisting of protein modules apparently derived from diverse protein families. The genes for C6, C7 and C9 are closely located on chromosome 5p13, while the genes for C8α and C8β are on the short arm of chromosome 1.

Inherited deficiencies of the terminal complement components have been reported to be frequently associated with recurrent systemic infections caused by *Neisseria meningitidis* or *Neisseria gonorrhoeae*: meningococcal meningitis, meningococcemia, and disseminated gonococcal infection, although C9-deficient individuals seem to be at much decreased risk of infection [1–3]. In this paper, we describe the studies performed for 16 years in our laboratory on the terminal complement component deficiencies in Japan, with emphasis on C9 deficiency (C9D).

A Large-Scale Screening of Complement Deficiencies in Japan

In order to determine the frequency of deficiency for each component of the complement system, a large-scale screening was performed [4, 5]. As a first step, a hemolytic assay

KARGER
Fax +41 61 306 12 34
E-Mail karger@karger.ch
www.karger.com

0254–9670/98/0154–0244$17.50/0

Accessible online at:
http://BioMedNet.com/karger

Yasuo Fukumori
Osaka Red Cross Blood Center
2-4-43, Morinomiya, Joto-ku, Osaka 536-8505 (Japan)
Tel. +81 6 962 7001, Fax +81 6 968 4900
E-Mail yfoichan@al.mbn.or.jp

(CH50) using sucrose-gelatin-Veronal buffer (SGVB) was carried out [4]. By using SGVB instead of the standard buffer, gelatin-Veronal buffer (GVB), we were able to increase the sensitivity in detecting C9D sera. By further examinations including hemolytic and protein assays of each of the components, component-deficient sera could be distinguished from sera with low CH50 activity caused by nonspecific activation of complement. Among 145,640 donors in the Osaka area (Japan), we found 2 cases with inherited C5D, 4 with C6D, 6 with C7D, 4 with C8 α-γ subunit deficiency (C8α-γD) and 138 with C9D with an indcidence of 0.0014, 0.0027, 0.0041, 0.0027 and 0.0948%, respectively [4, 5]. Hayama et al. [6] reported that among 92,686 sera from hospitalized patients throughout Japan, 80 were found to be deficient in C9 using the same screening system. The incidence of C9D nationwide was determined to be about 0.086%, and no significant differences were observed among the 8 areas of Japan tested [6]. It is concluded that the incidence of homozygous C9D is almost 1 in 1,000 in Japan. C2D, the most common deficiency in the Caucasian population, was not found in either of these two screenings. In spite of the high incidence of C9D and other terminal complement components, no deficiencies of the early components were identified in the Japanese population.

Reports on Complement Deficiencies from Hospitals in Japan

Additional cases with complement deficiencies have been reported from hospitals in Japan: 2 patients with C3D, 3 with C5D, 2 with C6D, 11 with C7D and 1 with C8α-γD. The frequency of C7D was supposed to be relatively high compared with those of C5D, C6D and C8α-γD in Japan (table 1). To establish the relation between the terminal component deficiencies including C9D in Japan and meningitis, we summed up the reported data on patients with meningitis in Japan [3]. The association with meningitis was observed in 2 cases with C6D, 9 with C7D and 9 with C9D.

Table 1. Total numbers of terminal complement component deficiencies reported in Japan, from 1981 to 1997

	C5D	C6D	C7D	C8D	C9D
Reports[1]	3	2	11	1	301[3]
Screening[2]	2	4	6	4	138
Total	5	6	17	5	439

1 Reports from hospitals throughout Japan.
2 From the screening [3, 4].
3 Including other screenings in [6], Fukuoka and Saitam (data not shown).

The results on the complement deficiencies in Japan support the existence of an ethnic predominance for C2D, C8α-γD, C8βD and C9D. C2D and C8γD were not identified in Japan, while C8α-γD and C9D, which are extremely rare in Caucasians, are not uncommon in Japan, especially C9D.

Molecular Basis of the Terminal Complement Component Deficiencies in Japan

Causes of complement component deficiencies are increasingly being investigated at the molecular level. However, the molecular genetic bases of the inherited deficiencies have not been determined except for C5D, C8βD and subtotal C6 deficiency until recently. Our group has elucidated the molecular genetic bases of some of the individuals with

Table 2. Molecular genetic analyses of complement deficiencies in Japan

Deficient in	Sample	Deficient allele
C6	1	one deletion at nt 291/unknown[1]
C7	1	two deletions at nt 2137-8 (homozygote)
	2	T→A transversion at nt 2250 (homozygote)
C8α–γ	1	g→t transversion at intron 2 (homozygote)
	2	g→t transversion at intron 2/C→T transition at exon 9
	3	g→a transition at intron 6/unknown
C9	1–8	C→T transition at nt 343 (homozygote)
	9	C→T transition at nt 343/G→A transition at nt 1580
	10	C→T transition at nt 343/unknown

[1] The putative mutation in the other deficient allele was not identified by our methods.

C6D, C7D, C8α-γD and C9D, using an exon-specific PCR-SSCP method followed by direct sequencing of the target exons [7–10].

One C6D Japanese had a heterozygous single base deletion (291, 292, 293 or 294delC) in exon 2 of the C6 gene [7]. However, the putative mutation in the other allele of the C6 gene remains unknown. Another C6D individual who is an African-American had a homozygous single base deletion at nucleotide (nt) 1936 (1936delG) [7]. Both mutations resulted in a frame shift and in the generation of a stop codon downstream.

In 2 unrelated C7D individuals, homozygous mutations in exon 16 of case 1 and in exon 15 of case 2 were identified [8]. The mutation of case 1 was a homozygous T→A transversion at nt 2250, the third nucleotide of the codon TGT for Cys 728, leading to a stop codon TGA (C728X). In case 2, a homozygous 2-bp deletion (2137delTG/2138delGT/2139delTG) caused a frame shift, generating a premature termination codon 4–6 nucleotides downstream. The analyses of 3 other C7D, 2 C7D Japanese and 1 Spanish are in progress. They have neither of the above two mutations.

In 3 unrelated Japanese C8α-γD individuals, we found 3 types of deficiency in the C8A gene, a splice junction mutation in exon 2/intron 2 boundary, a nonsense mutation in exon 9 [9], and a splice mutation in intron 6 [P.M. Schneider, pers. commun.]. The first mutation was homozygous in case 1 and heterozygous in case 2. The second was found to be heterozygous in case 2. The third was a heterozygous mutation in case 3. The putative mutation in the other deficient allele of the C8A gene in case 3 remains unknown.

In 10 unrelated C9D subjects, 8 of the 10 were homozygous for a C→T transition at nt 343, the first nucleotide of the codon for Arg 95, leading to a TGA stop codon (R95X). One of the 10 carried a compound heterozygous mutation consisting of the R95X and a G→A transition at nt 1580 that leads to the substitution of Cys 507→Tyr (C507Y). Another of the 10 was also heterozygous for the R95X mutation; however, the mutation on the other allele was not identified by our methods. R95X is thus identified in most cases of C9D in Japan (18 of 20 null alleles) [10]. The molecular bases for C9D in a Swiss family have been previously found to be a compound heterozygote for 2 nonsense mutations at nucleotide 166 and 464, a C→A transversion leading to a TGA stop codon (C33X), and a C→T transition leading to a TGA stop codon (R133X), respectively [11].

We summarize these results in table 2. These results suggest that the genetic bases of the C6D, C7D and C8D are heterogeneous whereas that of C9D is homogeneous, suggesting C9D is caused by a founder effect.

Predominance of the C9-Deficient Gene (R95X) in Asia

In order to directly prove that the R95X gene is really distributed in a general Japanese population at the DNA level, we examined the presence of the R95X gene in normal donors using a PCR-RFLP method with mismatch primers and *Bst*UI. We found 22 heterozygous individuals among 302 healthy persons in Japan. The incidence of the R95X gene (3.6%) is nearly identical to the predicted incidence of C9D (3.2%) calculated by the Hardy-Weinberg equation from the serological results in our large-scale screening. This concordance suggests that C9D in Japan is mostly caused by the R95X gene.

Furthermore, to establish where and when the R95X gene has originated, we examined DNA subjects from other ethnic groups (Ryukyuans, who are Japanese living in Southern islands, Koreans, Thais, Germans and Italians) using the PCR-RFLP method described above. We found considerable numbers of individuals carrying the R95X in all Asian populations but not in European populations [manuscript in preparation]. The Japanese, Ryukyuans and Koreans belong to the East Asians whereas the Thais belong to the South Asians. The R95X gene is supposed to have originated after the Caucasians and Mongoloids were divided and before East and South Asians were divided. As for C2D, which is common among Caucasians, there seems to be a founder effect for individuals with C9D among Asians.

Acknowledgments

We thank Drs. H. Kitamura (Osaka Prefecture College of Health Science), T. Amano (Okayama University), H. Nishizaka, T. Kojima (Kyushu University), H. Nishimukai (Ehime University), H. Shibata, Y. Okubo, K. Yoshimura (Osaka Red Cross Blood Center), P.M. Schneider (Johannes Gutenberg University Mainz, Germany) and F. Tedesco (University of Trieste, Italy) for supporting our studies.

References

1 Inai S, Kitamura H, Hiramatsu S, Nagaki K: Deficiency of the ninth component of complement in man. J Clin Lab Immunol 1979;2:85–87.

2 Kitamura H, Nagaki K, Inai S: Further studies on C9 deficiency. J Clin Lab Immunol 1981;6:7–11.

3 Nagata M, Hara T, Aoki T, Mizuno Y, Akeda H, Inaba S, Tsumoto K: Inherited deficiency of ninth component of complement: An increased risk of meningococcal meningitis. J Pediatr 1989;114:260–264.

4 Fukumori Y, Yoshimura K, Ohnoki S, Yamaguchi H, Akagaki Y, Inai S: A high incidence of C9 deficiency among healthy blood donors in Osaka, Japan. Int Immunol 1989;1:85–89.

5 Inai S, Akagaki Y, Moriyama T, Fukumori Y, Yoshimura K, Ohnoki S, Yamaguchi H: Inherited deficiencies of the late-acting complement components other than C9 found among healthy blood donors. Int Arch Allergy Appl Immunol 1989;90:274–279.

6 Hayama K, Sugai N, Tanaka S, Lee H, Kikuchi J, Ito J, Suzuki Y, Nagata H, Kondo H, Harayama K, Tuzuki S, Yoshida M, Fujita F, Ohmori T, Kawai Y, Akagaki Y, Inai S: High incidence of C9 deficiency throughout Japan: There are no significant differences in incidence among eight areas of Japan. Int Arch Allergy Appl Immunol 1989;9:400–404.
7 Nishizaka H, Horiuchi T, Zhu ZB, Fukumori Y, Ngasawa K, Hayashi K, Krumdieck R, Cobbs CG, Higuchi M, Yasunaga S, Volanakis JE: Molecular bases for inherited human complement component C6 deficiency in two unrelated individuals. J Immunol 1996;156:2309–2315.
8 Nishizaka H, Horiuchi T, Zhu ZB, Fukumori Y, Volanakis JE: Genetic bases of human complement C7 deficiency. J Immunol 1996;157:4239–4243.
9 Kojima T, Horiuchi T, Nishizaka H, Fukumori Y, Amano T, Nagasawa K, Niho Y, Hayashi K: Genetic basis of human complement C8α-γ deficiency. J Immunol 1998;161:3762–3766.
10 Horiuchi T, Nishizaka H, Kojima T, Sawabe T, Niho Y, Schneider PM, Inaba S, Sakai K, Hayashi K, Hashimura C, Fukumori Y: A non-sense mutation at Arg95 is predominant in complement 9 deficiency in Japanese. J Immunol 1998;160:1509–1513.
11 Witzel-Schlömp K, Späth PJ, Hobart MJ, Fernie BA, Rittner C, Kaufmann T, Schneider PM: The human complement C9 gene identification of two mutations causing deficiency and revision of the gene structure. J Immunol 1997;158:5043–5049.

Experimental and Clinical
Immunogenetics

Exp Clin Immunogenet 1998;15:249–260

Received: December 22, 1998
Accepted: December 29, 1998

G. Mauff[a]
Birgit Luther[a]
P.M. Schneider[b]
C. Rittner[b]
Beate Stradmann-Bellinghausen[b]
R. Dawkins[c]
Joann M. Moulds[d]

[a] Department Immunology, Virology, Vaccinations, State Institute of Hygiene, Hamburg,
[b] Institute of Legal Medicine, University of Mainz, Germany;
[c] Centre for Molecular Immunology and Instrumentation, University of Western Australia, Nedlands, Australia, and
[d] Division of Rheumatology and Clinical Immunogenetics, University of Texas Medical School, Houston, Tex., USA

Reference Typing Report for Complement Component C4

Key Words
Complement genetics
C4
Reference typing
*Taq*I RFLP
Rodgers/Chido PCR

Abstract

During the 7th Complement Genetics Workshop, Mainz, Germany, May 1998, a complement component C4 typing exercise took place with the aim of applying present technologies to the definition of *reference C4 alleles/phenotypes* and the recognition of nonexpressed (Q0) C4 alleles within expressed haplotypes. Eleven samples were submitted from 3 laboratories and tested by 14 participating laboratories with basic protein-typing technologies; in addition, each laboratory contributed data from local expertise. The samples were introduced to the reference typing for one or more characteristic allotype or for partial or total nonexpression of one isotype. The blinded samples were centrally evaluated and the results discussed among the participants at a plenum meeting. From the results, the samples could be classified into a group of common, easy to diagnose pheno-/allotypes, less common but still unanimously recognised variants, and a third group with difficult pheno-/allotypes. Within the latter group, the allotypes were either new (C4A '92'; C4B '93') and/or showed partial or total reversed antigenicity and unusual Rodgers/Chido (Rg/Ch) PCR subtypes (C4A '92'; C4A 12; C4B '35'; C4B '13'). Semiquantitative C4-α-chain estimates of relative isotype levels correlated well with the number of alleles seen at each locus by agarose gel electrophoresis, and were superior to other isotype quantitation methods. From the evaluation of the reference typing it was concluded that the recognition of rare, aberrant or hybrid C4 alleles with partial or total reversed Rg/Ch antigenicity or monoclonal reactivity is still difficult in most instances; besides isotype-dependent lysis, relative migration values, immunoblots with Rg- and Ch-specific monoclonal antibodies, Rg/Ch PCR typing, side-by-side comparison with already described allotypes will ultimately be required. The recognition of nonexpressed alleles within C4A and C4B expressed phenotypes remains the major obstacle in C4 genetic typing. Finally, a conclusive interpretation of DNA typing results will be achieved only in the context of complete allotyping results at the protein level, and at present cannot replace conventional protein allotyping.

In commemoration of Prof. Tomi Meo (†)

On behalf of: G. Arason, Reykjavik, Iceland; I. Berkel, Ankara, Turkey; M. Brai, Palermo, Italy; M. Cuccia, Pavia, Italy; M. Lokki, Helsinki, Finland; E. Paz-Artal, Madrid, Spain; P. Santos, Coimbra, Portugal; L. Truedsson, Lund, Sweden; L. Weiss, Paris, France; Y. Yu, Columbus, Ohio, USA.

KARGER

Fax + 41 61 306 12 34
E-Mail karger@karger.ch
www.karger.com

0254–9670/98/0154–0249$17.50/0

Accessible online at:
http://BioMedNet.com/karger

Prof. G. Mauff, Hygiene Institut Hamburg
Abteilung Immunologie, Virologie und Impfwesen
Marckmannstrasse 129a, D–20539 Hamburg (Germany)
Tel. +49 40 42837 235, Fax +49 40 42837 482
E-Mail hyginsthh@vossnet.de

Introduction

Since the first discovery of complete deficiency of the fourth human complement component (C4) [1], localization of the C4 genes within the major histocompatibility complex [2–4], and description of the technology for the determination of genetic C4 polymorphism [5, 6], C4 has proven to be among the most complex complement and plasma proteins. Subsequent studies resulted in further insight into the relationship between Rodgers (Rg) and Chido (Ch) antigens and C4 [7–9], the genomic organization of C4, duplication of its structural genes and very close linkage with the 21-hydroxylase genes [4, 10, 11], and on the molecular basis for the functional difference between the two isotypes, C4A and C4B [12–14]. Nevertheless, on a methodological basis, the complete allotyping of the large number of alleles, recognition of gene duplications, nonexpressions and deletions have resisted easy approaches.

Reference typing exercises have therefore been performed previously for the allotyping of the multiple genetic variants of C4 [15, 16]. Alleles were characterized by comparison of electrophoretic migration, characterization of hemolytic activity, reactivity with isotype-specific monoclonal antibodies, and presence of Rg and Ch epitopes. In addition, classification of C4α- and β-chains and correlation of protein data with *Taq*I RFLP patterns on the genomic level to identify duplicated and nonexpressed (Q0) C4 genes were attempted [17–19]. They have resulted in several reference typing reports and C4 nomenclature statements [15, 16, 20–23].

For the classification of C4 alleles, their relative electrophoretic mobility in a defined buffer system, the difference in hemolytic activity of isotypes, correlating with the presence or absence of the Ch4 antigen, and determination of Rg/Ch-specific DNA sequences as recognized by PCR [24, 25] are now the major criteria of definition. Allotypes may further be subdivided according to parameters derived from the aforementioned methods. The reference typings have resulted in the description of more than 23 C4A and 26 C4B allotypes until today [26].

It has been the aim of C4 reference typing during the 7th Complement Genetics Workshop, Mainz, Germany, May 1998, to apply present technologies to the definition of *reference C4 alleles/phenotypes* and recognition of C4 Q0 within expressed haplotypes with the ultimate goal of achieving international standardization. The procedures, results and conclusions are reported here.

Materials and Methods

Eleven samples as listed in table 1 were submitted from laboratories in Mainz, Hamburg, and Houston, Tex., and were distributed to all participating laboratories. These were represented by: G. Arason, Reykjavik; I. Berkel, Ankara; M. Brai, Palermo; M. Cuccia, Pavia; R. Dawkins, Perth; M. Lokki, Helsinki; G. Mauff, Hamburg; J. Moulds, Houston; E. Paz-Artal, Madrid; P. Santos, Coimbra; P. Schneider, Mainz; L. Truedsson, Lund; L. Weiss, Paris; Y. Yu, Columbus. Besides the basic protein technology, each laboratory contributed data from additional local expertise. The typing methods, as summarized in table 2, included all presently used technologies for C4 characterization with the exception of Rg/Ch serotyping.

Most samples were submitted for reference typing of one or more characteristic allotypes or partial or total nonexpression of one isotype. All of them were known to the submitting laboratory and had been characterized by various methods on different occasions. Two samples (DG25, BSB) were included because of previous difficulties in their allotypic interpretation.

Coded EDTA plasma samples and extracted DNA were aliquotted and stored at –70 °C in the submitting laboratories until shipment on dry ice to the participating laboratories. Sample AR15 was communicated as C4A 3, B 1 and used as reference phenotype and calibrator. AR15 has been in use as a standard for more than 18 years and participated in all previous reference exercises.

The typing technologies are summarized in table 1. C4 allotyping by high-voltage agarose gel electrophoresis with subsequent immunofixation on neuraminidase- and carboxypeptidase-treated samples was the basic procedure required from all participants. Further test parameters were reported according to special expertise of the individual laboratories. C4 activity from hemolytic overlays was tested by 6 participants, immunoblots with monoclonal antibodies by 7 laboratories, C4 isotype or total protein level by 3 laboratories.

DNA typing of the reference samples was carried out by 6 laboratories using RFLP analysis of *Taq*I-digested genomic DNA to determine the number of C4 genes, and by direct PCR typing of the DNA sequence polymorphisms giving rise to the Rg and Ch antigenic determinants. In the course of this collaborative exercise, it was observed that the names of two primer pairs were erroneously exchanged in the original publication by Barba et al. [24]: the sequence of primer Ch–5 has to be exchanged with the sequence of primer Ch+5, and the sequence of primer Rg3 has to be exchanged with the sequence of primer Ch6.

One of the organizing laboratories supplied C4-α-chain data, another laboratory supplied relative migration (RM) values, and two laboratories supplied HLA-B-DRB and -DQA/B PCR typing results.

All data sheets on the blinded samples were centrally evaluated by the organizing laboratories and the results discussed at a plenum meeting of the reference exercise participants during the 7th Workshop. Unanimous results were found on 6 reference type samples, differing results on 5 samples. They will be discussed in more detail in the following section.

Results

The investigated samples could be classified into three groups of common, easy to diagnose phenotypes/allotypes, less common but still unanimously recognised variants, and a third group with difficult phenotypes/allotypes which will be discussed in more detail (fig. 2). The data from the different participating laboratories were very satisfactory as concerns comparability of allotyping results from immunofixation and hemolysis in general (table 2). This was true also for *Taq*I RFLP determinations and, to a lesser extent, for Rg1 and Ch1 PCR results. Significant discrepancies were observed for the isotype-specific quantitations as compared between total, EIA and densitometric plasma levels, especially in samples DG25, XR, BSB, and NBW. However, considering that by EIA the total of antigenic determinants recognised by one monoclonal antibody, including those variants with partial or total reversed antigenicity, were determined as compared to isotype attribution on electrophoretic separations according to monoclonal reactivity on immunoblots, the isotype concentrations were still in comparable dimensions. Total C4 levels were higher throughout by radial immunodiffusion from laboratory 1, but followed the same tendency as in laboratory 2 and EIA results. C4α-chain typing provided a semiquantitative estimate of relative amounts for C4A versus C4B α-chains and correlated well with the number of alleles recognized for each locus and isotype by agarose gel electrophoresis and subsequent immunofixation and lysis.

The densitometric determination of RM values [16] was done on 10 different immunofixation agarose gel electrophoreses (9 separations for BS), calibrated with sample AR15: reference distance C4B 1→A 3 = 100 and the means and standard deviations calculated as shown in table 2. The mean RM values for all C4A 3, B 1 (except the calibrator) was 102.2, for all C4A 4, B 1 109.4, thus sufficiently close to previously published values [20, 26, 27]. Not all other variants met the requirements of the mean lying within the range of reported variants or vice versa, as limited by the precision of the method. However, on the grounds of multiple preceding determinations, monoclonal antibody reactivity, Rg/Ch PCR types and *Taq*I fragments in sample DG25 C4B 6, in XR C4B 2, in GR C4B 5, in BSB C4A 6 and 55 in BS C4A 12 were regarded as congruent with C4 nomenclature standards. With DG25, one unusual allele was seen, designat-

Table 1. Methods of C4 reference typing, 1998

Methods	Conditions	References
1. C4 allotyping		
Buffer system	Tris-glycine-barbital	6
Neuraminidase	*C. perfringens* type VI (Sigma)	15, 16
Carboxypeptidase B	type I (Sigma)	
Electrophoretic conditions	3–4 h, 400–800 V (alt. 70–90 mA const.)	
Type/source of antibodies	anti-C4 goat IgG (Biogenesis; Quidel)	
Hemolytic overlay	C4-deficient guinea pig serum	
Western blot (MAB)	99H7, 1228, RGd1(Rg1), Ch1(O33C-30.27), Ch3	
2. C4α-chain typing		
SDS-PAGE of immuno-precipitated serum C4	10% T, 0.06% C denaturing SDS-polyacrylamide gel	17, 23
Protein staining	Kenacid blue protein staining	
Type/source of antibodies (Western blot)	anti-C4 goat IgG (Quidel) for immunoprecipitation, MAB for detection as above	
3. Relative migration		
	densitometry (Gel-Doc 1000 Bio-Rad) software molecular analyst / PC	27
4. Rodgers/Chido antigens		
Serology	Plasma inhibition / hemagglutination	21
Type/source of antisera/antibodies	Human polyclonal antisera, MAB as in 1	
PCR typing	C4 isotype-specific primers: A-up/down, B-up/down Rg/Ch sequence-specific primers: Rg1, Rg3, Ch1, Ch-5, Ch5, Ch6	24, 25
5. C4A/B quantitation		
Methods	EIA radial immunodiffusion, densitometry	28, 29, 30
Source/type of antisera	Partigen (Chiron Behring), MAB as in 1	
6. C4 Taq*I RFLP*		
Method	Agarose gel electrophoresis of *Taq*I-digested genomic DNA, followed by Southern blotting, hybridization with C4- and CYP21-specific DNA probes and autoradiography	19, 22
C4 probe	500-bp *Bam*HI/*Kpn*I fragment of C4 cDNA clone pAT-A	31
CYP21 probe	900-bp *Bg*lI fragment of genomic cosmid clone 1E3	11
7. HLA typing		
PCR	B, SSP Biosynthesis Kit, in-house method, DRB: SSO Kit, Dynal RELI SSO DRB typing kit DQA, B	32, 33, 34

ed from earlier typing results as C4B 3. In further determinations during this workshop it did not fit B 3 and has now been renamed 'B 35', as an aberrant allele with partially reversed antigenicity (Rg1+, Ch1–, 3–, see table 2). Since side-by-side comparison with adjacent variant alleles was not possible, the designation was tentative, with quotation marks. A second unusual allele, 'B 13', was observed for the first time in the same individual during this workshop. By RM measurement, this allele might also be a 'B 14', so far not described, but adjacent variants were not available at the workshop for comparison. Isotype assignment by lysis proved to be difficult because of close migration anodal to B 1. From previous family studies, the haplotype had been assumed to be HLA-Bw55, C4A 4, B 6, *Taq*I 7.0, 5.4, C4β HH, DRw6 [35]. With presently available information, a complete

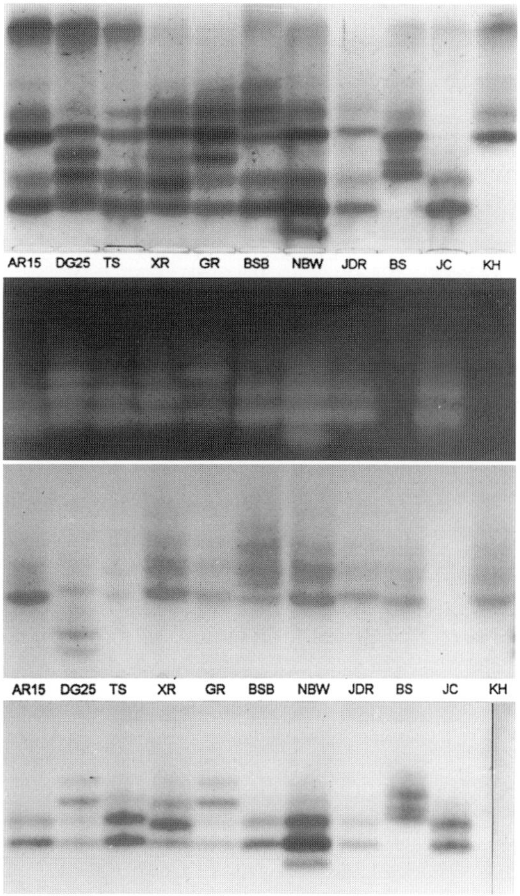

Fig. 1. C4 reference variant phenotyping by agarose gel electrophoresis. **a** Immunofixation with polyclonal anti-C4. **b** Hemolytic overlay containing C4-deficient guinea pig serum. **c** Immunoblot with monoclonal anti-C4A (MAB 99H7). **d** Immunoblot with monoclonal anti-C4B (MAB 1228).

Sample	Ethnic origin	Phenotype	
		C4A	C4B
AR15	caucasoid	3	1
DG25	caucasoid	4	6,'35','13',1
TS	caucasoid	3	1
XR	mongoloid	4	2,1
GR	caucasoid	4,3	5,1
BSB	caucasoid	6,55,3	1
NBW	caucasoid	3	1,'93'
JDR	caucasoid	4	1
BS	negroid	3,12[1],'92'	Q0
JC	caucasoid	Q0	1
KH	caucasoid	3	Q0

1 Aberrant or hybrid allotypes with partially or totally reversed antigenicity; allotypes in quotation marks are either newly detected or not finally assigned.

haplotype assignment of the 'B 13' allele will not be possible.

Sample NBW was first estimated to possess the slow C4B 92 allotype. On the basis of repeated RM determinations, this allele was found to migrate in between B 92 and 94 but to be distinct from both; it was therefore designated B '93' (new) pending side-by-side comparison.

Protein allotyping of sample BS also proved to be difficult. There were 3 prominent bands (fig. 1), all of isotype C4A by lysis, but 2 of them with aberrant antigenicity on immunoblots. From RM measurements the alleles were diagnosed as C4A '92', C4A 12 and the common C4A 3. A '92' was distinct in RM values from A 91 and therefore tentatively introduced pending future side-by-side comparison with a C4A 92 variant described earlier [36] but never defined in a reference exercise. A 4th band migrating in the position of C4A 2 was considered to be the minor band of A '92' since only 3 alleles appear to be expressed from C4α-chains and *Taq*I RFLP.

The RFLP results are shown in figure 2 and summarized in table 2, column 9, and are consistent with the C4 allotyping results in most samples. Deletions of C4/CYP21 gene pairs were observed in samples TS, JDR, BS and JC. In JDR and JC, both a C4A/CYP21A

Table 2. C4 and MHC typing data of reference variants

[1]Samples	[2]C4 allotypes	[3]RM	[4]Lysis type	[5]Antigenicity (MAB: IB, EIA)	[6]Rg/Ch antigens Rg	[6]Rg/Ch antigens Ch	[6]Rg/Ch PCR subtype	[7]C4α-chains
AR 15	A 3,3	(100)	A	A	1		0301	Aα: 4
	B 1,1	0	B	B		1	0101	Bα: 5
DG 25	A 4, Q0	109.6 (±4.8)	A	A	1		0401	Aα: 1
	B 6	74.2 (±1.6)	B	B		1	0601	Bα: 6
	B '35'	43.8 (±1.7)	B	A	1		3503	
	B '13'	15.2 (±2.7)	(B?)	A	1		1303	
	B 1	0	B	B		1	0101	
TS	A 3, Q0	102.4 (±2.2)	A	A	1		0301	Aα: 3
	B 1,1	0	B	B		1	0101	Bα: 7
XR	A 4,(4)	106.5 (±1.7)	A	A	1		0401	Aα: 3
	B 2	31.6 (±1.4)	B	B		1	0201	Bα: 5
	B 1	0	B	B		1	0101	
GR	A 4	111.6 (±3.9)	A	A	1		0401	Aα: 3
	A 3	100.0 (±2.0)	A	A	1		0301	Bα: 5
	B 5	70.1 (±1.8)	B	B		1	0501/5	
	B 1	0	B	B		1	0105/1	
BSB	A 6	142.4 (±3.8)	A	A	1		0601	Aα: 5
	A 55	126.1 (±4.9)	A	A	1		5501	Bα: 6
	A 3	101.5 (±2.2)	A	A	1		0301	
	B 1	0	B	B		1	0101	
	B 1	0	B	B		1	0102	
NBW	A 3,3	104.9 (±2.4)	A	A	1		0301	Aα: 2
	B 1,1	0	B	B		1	0101	Bα: 5
	B '93'	–35.6 (±1.4)	B	B		1	9302	
JDR	A 4, Q0	110.3 (±4.3)	A	A	1		0401	Aα: 2
	B 1, Q0	0	B	B		1	0101	Bα: 4
BS	A 3	(100) n.d.	A	A	1		0302/6	Aα: 6
	A 12	60.7 (±2.5)	A	B		1	1203/7	Bα: 0
	A '92'	43.2 (±3.0)	A	B		1	9203/7	
	B Q0	–	–	–			Q0	
JC	A Q0	–	–	–			Q0	Aα: 0
	B 1	0	B	B		1	0101	Bα: 6
KH	A 3,3	(100) n.d.	A	A	1		0301	Aα: 6
	B Q0	–	–	–			Q0	Bα: 0

1 For origin of samples, see table 3.
2 Allotype nomenclature according to ref. 15, 20.
3 RM units from standard immunofixation electrophoresis (table 1, 3.), mean values from 10 determinations using AR15 (B1 $\rightarrow$ A3 = 100 units) as calibration distance, in sample BS only 9 values for A '92' were available; n.d. = not determined.
4 Hemolytic activity as in table 1, 1; B '13' too close to B 1 to judge definitely type of lysis.
5 IB = Immunoblot; EIA = enzyme immuno assay; both with monoclonal antibodies (table 1, 1.).
6 Rg/Ch numbers refer to detectable antigens by IB using MAB 99H7 and 1228. In individual GR and BS assignment of Rg/Ch PCR subtype inconclusive, as both Ch+5 and Ch–5 have been detected. Thus, assignments cannot be made to a specific allele without family studies; for PCR subtype nomenclature, see ref. 25.
7 Intensity of C4α-chain bands from 1 (= weak) to 6 (very strong); 0 = no band detectable.

[8]C4 quantitation, mg/dl				[9]*Taq*I fragments, kb		[10]BF, IEF PCR	[11]HLA			
C4	D	EIA	RID	C4A/CYP21A	C4B/CYP21B		B	DR	DQA	DQB
A	15.4	18.1		a) 7.0/3.2	6.0/3.7	F, F	7,58	8,13	n.d.	n.d.
B	19.2	20.2		b) 7.0/3.2+	5.4+/3.7	FA, FA				
Total			L3: 52.5, L1: 34.6							
A	17.3	10.5		a) 7.0/3.2	5.4/3.7	S07, S	27,55	4,14	n.d.	n.d.
B	11.9	21.1		b) 7.0/3.2	5.4+/3.7+	S, S				
Total			L3: 39.1, L1: 29.2							
A	4.2	6.5		a) 7.0/3.2	6.0/3.7	S, S	8,44	3,7	n.d.	n.d.
B	17.9	18.9		b) –/–	6.4/3.7	S, S				
Total			L3: 30.0, L1: 22.2							
A	9.6	14.5		a) 7.0/3.2	5.4/3.7	F, S	55,37	8,10	n.d.	n.d.
B	16.5	14.6		b) 7.0/3.7	5.4/3.7	FB, S				
Total			L3: 36.0, L1: 26.1	or: 7.0/–	–/3.7					
A	5.0	7.7		a) 7.0/3.2	6.0/3.7	S, S	7,35	2,4	n.d.	n.d.
B	16.4	15.4		b) 7.0/3.2	5.4/3.7	S, S				
Total			L3: 30.0, L1: 21.4							
A	8.3	20.5		a) 7.0/3.2	6.0/3.7	F, S	51,57	2,7	n.d.	n.d.
B	18.1	13.8		b) 7.0/3.2	5.4+/3.7+	FA, S				
Total			L3: 36.0, L1: 26.4							
A	15.3	23.6		a) 7.0/3.2	5.4/3.7	F, S	13,44	7	0501	0201
B	34.4	26.0		b) 7.0/3.2+	5.4+/3.7	FB, S			0201	0201
Total			L3: 67.5, L1: 49.7							
A	3.7	4.2		a) 7.0/–	–/3.7	S, S	8,X	3,14	0501	0201
B	6.3	6.8		b) –/–	6.4/3.7	S, S			0104	0503
Total			L3: 14.4, L1: 10.0							
A	9.6	5.2		a) 7.0/3.2	5.4/3.7	F1, F	7,15	3,X	0401	0201
B	10.6	17.3		b) 7.0/–	–/3.7	S, FB			0501	0402
Total			L3:27.7, L1: 20.2							
A	–	–		a) 7.0/–	–/3.7	S, S	8,X	3,X	0101	0301
B	17.6	14.6		b) –/–	6.4/3.7	S, S			0501	0201
Total			L3: 23.1, L1: 17.6							
A	19.4	18.0		a) 7.0/3.2	6.0/3.7	F, S	35,65	7,13	0201	0201
B	–	–		b) 7.0/3.2	6.0/3.7	FA, S			0103	0603
Total			L3: 25.8, L1: 19.4							

8 D = from relative densitometric evaluation of immunofixation electrophoresis and RID (table 2) from Lab 1; EIA (table 2); RID = radial immunodiffusion. C4A/B assignment of bands in densitometry according to MAB reactivity on IB; in RID total C4 plasma concentrations from laboratories 1 (L1) and 3 (L2). For reversed antigenicity, see text.

9 *Taq*I-RFLP results refer to detectable fragment sizes in kilobase pairs. CYP21A and B = 21-hydroxylase A and B genes. A '+' indicates a duplication of the respective gene. DNA haplotypes a) and b) are not assigned to defined C4 protein allo- or haplotypes. In sample XR, the presence of a possible CYP21A/C4B gene deletion is not yet confirmed (see 'Results').

10 Factor B (BF) phenotypes as determined by IEF (top) and PCR (bottom) in several laboratories; for technology, see ref. 37.

11 HLA B/DR typing by SSP and/or SS0 communicated by one laboratory, DRB/DQA-B subtypes by a second laboratory; X refers to second antigen or homozygosity; n.d. = not determined.

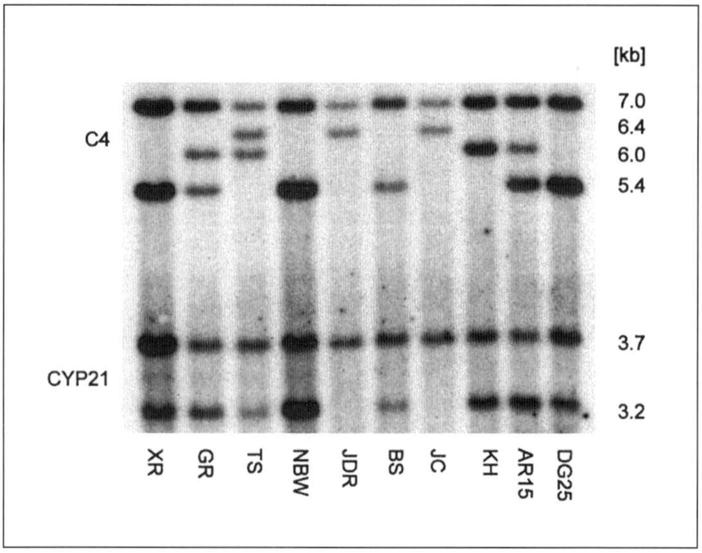

Fig. 2. C4/21-hydroxylase *Taq*I RFLP of workshop samples; for further characterization of samples, see table 1 and figure 1. BSB is not shown (RFLP type 7.0/3.2. 6.0/3.7 – 7.0/0.2, 5.4/3.7, see table 2).

and a C4B/CYP21B gene pair was missing, resulting in the presence of a single expressed C4A and B gene in JDR, and only a single C4B gene expressed in JC together with a copy of a nonexpressed C4A Q0 gene. The presence of this silent gene was confirmed by detecting a C4A-specific PCR amplification product without obtaining a corresponding C4A protein band by allotyping.

In two samples, the results were not conclusive in comparison to the protein typing results: in AR15, C4 allotyping, C4α-chains and ELISA results suggest a balanced expression of C4A and B alleles, whereas the *Taq*I results clearly demonstrate the presence of a CYP21A/short-C4B gene duplication. Thus, it may be assumed that one of the C4B genes could be nonexpressed. In XR, there is a clearly more intensive 3.7-kb CYP21B fragment, whereas the C4-specific 7.0- and 5.4-kb bands are almost equally strong (fig. 2, left lane). The results from ELISA and densitometry also indicate a balanced expression of the isotypes. Thus the intensive 3.7-kb fragment could be due to a rare gene conversion event changing CYP21A to CYP21B, or to a point mutation affecting the *Taq*I restriction site usually generating the 3.2-kb *Taq* fragment. Alternatively, a CYP21A/C4B gene deletion has to be assumed to explain this observation (see corresponding row for XR in table 2). In KH, it can be demonstrated that both copies of the (long) C4B genes have been converted completely to C4A, as only the C4A3 allotype can be detected at the protein level, and C4 PCR results indicate that only the C4A-specific primers generate an amplification product. C4 gene duplications could be detected in DG25, BSB, and NBW, and could be confirmed by identifying a corresponding number of C4A and/or C4B alleles.

The Rg/Ch PCR subtypes are summarized in table 2, last column 6. The four-digit nomenclature is composed of two sources: the first two digits represent the protein allotype as defined by immunofixation agarose gel electrophoresis, and the last two digits represent the genotypic combination of the Rg and Ch sequence epitopes according to a numerical system devised by Schneider et al. [25].

Table 3. Characteristics of the 7th Workshop C4 reference allotypes

Allotype	RM	Isotype lysis	mAb type 99H7	mAb type 1228	Rg/Ch PCR type	Reference samples	Origin
A Q0	–	–	–	–	–	JC	Houston
A 6	142	A	+	–	0601	BSB	Mainz
A 55	126	A	+	–	5501	BSB	Mainz
A 4	109[1]	A	+	–	0401	DG25/XR/JDR	Hamburg/Mainz/Houston
A 3	102[1]	A	+	–	0301	TS/NBW/KH	Hamburg/Mainz/Houston
A 12	61	A	–	+[2]	1203/7	BS	Houston
A '92'	43	A	–	+[2]	9103/7	BS	Houston
B Q0	–	–	–	–	–	KH	Houston
B 6	74	B	–	+	0601	DG25	Hamburg
B 5	70	B	–	+	0501/5	GR	Mainz
B '35'	44	B	+[2]	–	0303	DG25	Hamburg
B 2	32	B	–	+	0201	XR	Mainz
B '13'	15	B	+[2]	–	1103	DG25	Hamburg
B 1	0	B	–	+	0101	all[3]	Hamburg/Mainz/Houston
B '93'	36	B	–	+	9302	NBW	Houston

RM values from table 2 rounded to the nearest single unit; MAB = anti-Rg1 (99H7); anti-Ch1 (1228).
1 Mean of 40 determinations from 4 individuals of each allotype.
2 Antigenicity partially or totally reversed to isotype.
3 All samples except BS and KH.

PCR subtypes other than '01' were detected in samples DG25, GR, BSB, NBW, and BS. In DG25, BSB, and NBW, the assignment was supported by the results of Western blot analysis indicating the presence of a Rg1 epitope in a C4B allele. In GR and BS, a polymorphism was observed regarding the presence or absence of the Ch5 determinant in either C4B or C4A, respectively, which could not be conclusively assigned to a specific allele. Therefore, the alternative subtypes are listed in table 2, column 6, e.g. 0501/5, 0105/1 for GR. These subtypes can only be correctly identified in family studies or by Western blot analysis using Ch5-specific antiserum.

A summary of all relevant reference allotype characteristics will be found in table 3.

Conclusions

From the evaluation of the 7th Workshop C4 reference typing results, the following conclusions may be drawn:

(1) The allotyping of common C4 variants/phenotypes at the expression level is established and no major obstacles will be encountered by experienced laboratories with technologies described here. In principle, this also holds true for less common alleles, although the differentiation between C4A 3 and A 4, or the combination of A 4, 3 versus A 3 or A 4 in the single, unrelated individual may be more difficult, depending on the quality of electrophoretic separation. Other less common alleles, such as A 6, A 2, A 91, B 5, B 3, or B 2, will be recognised by their known linkage disequi-

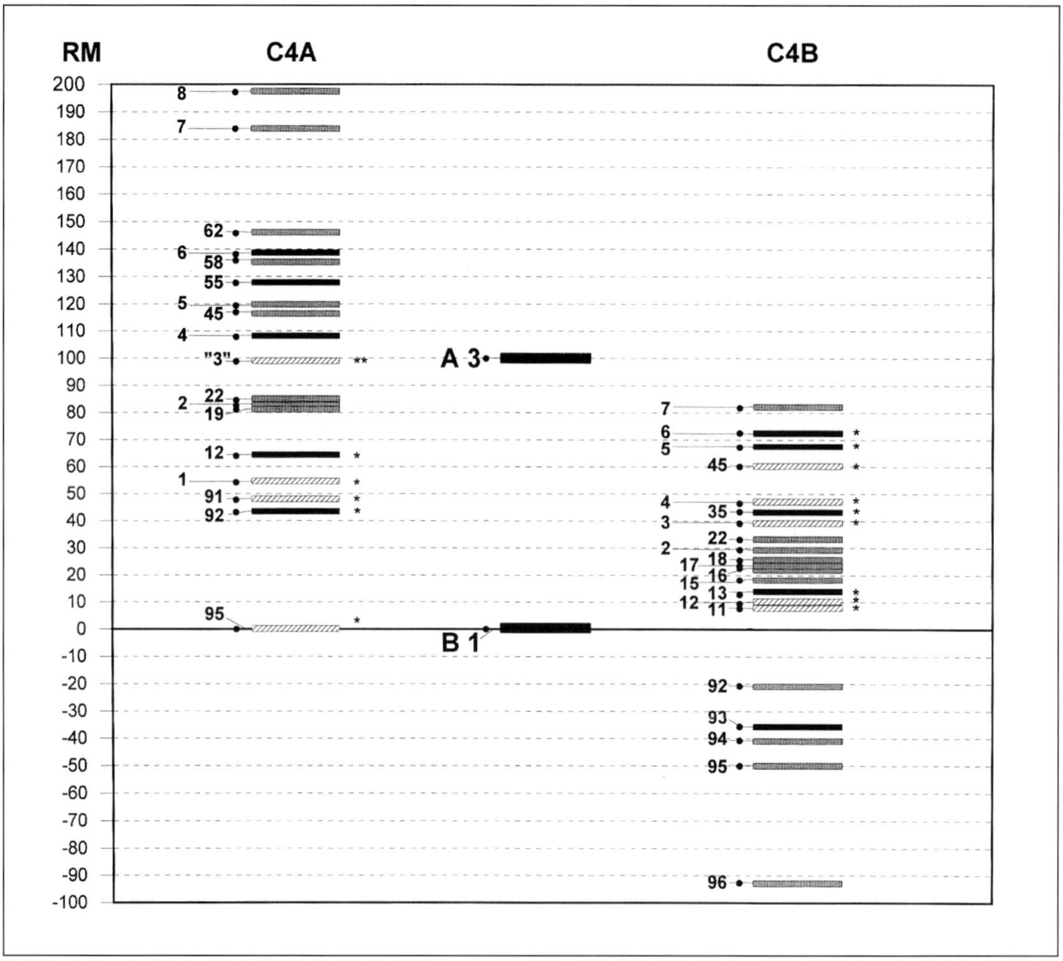

Fig. 3. Relative migration (RM) distances of 7th Workshop C4 reference variants (bold banding pattern) and of formerly defined C4 allotypes (actual RM positions marked by black dots.) * = RM positions, for which aberrant/hybrid alleles with partially or totally reversed antigenicity have been described [see ref. 26]. ** = Hybrid allele with C4A and C4B mAb reactivity [see ref. 38].

librium, by comparison with reference sera or determination of their relative migration.

The recognition of rarer, aberrant or hybrid alleles with partially or totally reversed Rg/Ch antigenicity or monoclonal reactivity has proven more difficult in most instances; besides isotype identification by lysis, it will require the determination of RM values, immunoblots with Rg- and Ch-specific monoclonal antibodies and essentially Rg/Ch-PCR typing, as well. Ultimately, the side-by-side comparison with already described allotypes should be the criterion for final classification in many instances. The RM positions of reference variants of this workshop, in comparison to formerly described C4 variants, will be found in figure 3.

(2) The recognition of nonexpressed (Q0) alleles within C4A and C4B expressed phenotypes was also attempted during this work-

shop. It still remains the major obstacle in C4 genetic typing. Quantitation of expressed isotype proteins by densitometry and EIA has now reached improved congruency, but is far from satisfactory in phenotypes with rare, duplicated or aberrant alleles; the semiquantitation of C4α-chains still seems superior to the other two methods if evaluated together with *Taq*I RFLP fragment patterns. However, the densitometric estimate from immunofixation electrophoresis gels has the advantage over all other methods to offer additional information without any further complex technology provided scanning facilities are available.

(3) A conclusive interpretation of DNA typing results can be achieved only in the context of complete allotyping results at the protein level, and at present cannot replace conventional protein allotyping. It may, however, provide useful partial information regarding structural C4 polymorphism as well as about point mutation and gene conversion events. In combination with C4 allotyping results, confirmation regarding the number of expressed genes can be obtained, and additional subtypes of protein allotypes may further be defined, increasing the complexity of C4 polymorphism.

(4) MHC linkage data, especially with HLA-B, DR/DQ and BF, may also be useful in the interpretation of C4 haplotypes if information from family studies is available. In the context of the present reference typing, family data were only known for some of the included individuals; no significant additional information was therefore obtained from this part of the investigation but may be necessary if some of the samples are to be defined in more detail in the future.

Acknowledgments

For technical, photographic and secretarial assistance, the authors are especially grateful to Mrs. Martina Bischof, Mrs. Anke Ebert, Mrs. Sigrid Glanschneider, Mrs. Ulrike Krause, Mrs. Sonja Scheunemann, and Mrs. Martina Wolke.

References

1 Hauptmann G, Grosshans E, Heid E: Lupus érythémateux aigu et déficit héréditaire en complément. A propos d'un cas par déficit complet en C4. Ann Derm Syph (Paris). 1974;101:479–496.
2 Rittner C, Hauptmann G, Grosse-Wilde H, Grosshans E, Tongio MM, Mayer S: Linkage between HLA (major histocompatibility complex) and genes controlling the synthesis of the fourth component of complement in Kissmeyer-Nielsen F (ed): Histocompatibility Testing. Heidelberg, Springer, 1975, p 945.
3 O'Neill GJ: Two HLA-linked loci controlling the fourth component of human complement. Proc Natl Acad Sci USA 1978;75:5165–5169.
4 Carroll MC, Campbell RD, Bentley DR, Porter RR: A molecular map of the human major histocompatibility complex class III region linking complement genes C4, C2 and factor B. Nature 1984;307:237–241.
5 Mauff G, Bender K, Fischer B: Genetic polymorphism of the fourth component of human complement. Vox Sang 1978;34:296–301.
6 Awdeh ZL, Alper CA: Inherited structural polymorphism of the fourth component of human complement. Proc Natl Acad Sci USA 1980;77:3576–3580.
7 Tilley CA, Romans DG, Crookston MC: Localization of Chido and Rodgers determinants to the C4d fragment of human C4. Nature 1978;276:713.
8 Giles CM, Batchelor JR, Dodi IA, Fiedler AHL, Rittner C, Mauff G, Bender K, Levene C, Schreuder GMTh, Wells LJ: C4 and HLA haplotypes associated with partial inhibition of anti-Rg and anti-Ch. Immunogenetics 1984;11:305–317.
9 Yu CY, Campbell RD, Porter RR: A structural model for the location of the Rodgers and the Chido antigenic determinants and their correlation with the human complement component C4A/C4B isotypes. Immunogenetics 1988;27:399–405.
10 Yu CY, Belt KT, Giles CM, Campbell RD, Porter RR: Structural basis of the polymorphism of human complement components C4A and C4B: Gene size, reactivity and antigenicity. EMBO J 1986;5:2873–2881.

11 Carroll MC, Palsdottir A, Belt KT, Porter RR: Deletion of complement C4 and steroid 21-hydroxylase genes in the HLA class III region. EMBO J 1985;4:2547–2552.
12 Isenman DE, Young JR: The molecular basis for the difference in immune hemolysis activity of the Chido and Rodgers isotypes of human complement component C4. J Immunol 1984;132:3019–3027.
13 Schifferli JA, Paccaud JP: Two isotypes of human C4, C4A and C4B have different structure and function. Complement Inflamm 1989;6: 19–26.
14 Carroll MC, Fathallah DM, Bergamaschini L, Alicot E, Isenman DE: Substitution of a single amino acid (aspartic acid for histidine) converts the functional activity of human complement C4B to C4A. Proc Natl Acad Sci USA 1990;87:6868–6872.
15 Mauff G, Alper CA, Awdeh Z, Batchelor JR, Bertrams J, Bruun-Petersen G, Dawkins RL, Demant P, Edwards J, Grosse-Wilde H, Hauptmann G, Klouda P, Lamm L, Mollenhauer E, Nerl C, Olaisen B, O'Neill G, Rittner C, Roos MH, Skanes V, Teisberg P, Wells L: Statement on the nomenclature of human C4 allotypes. Immunobiology 1983; 164:184–191.
16 Mauff G, Brenden M, Braun-Stilwell M, Doxiadis G, Giles C, Hauptmann G, Rittner C, Schneider PM, Stradmann-Bellinghausen B, Uring-Lambert B: C4 reference typing report. Complement Inflamm 1990;7: 193–212.
17 Roos MH, Mollenhauer E, Demant P, Rittner C: A molecular basis for the two locus model of human complement component C4. Nature 1982;298:854–856.
18 Mauff G, Steuer M, Weck M, Bender K: The C4β-chain: Evidence for a genetically determined polymorphism. Hum Genet 1983;64:186–188.
19 Schneider PM, Carroll MC, Alper CA, Rittner C, Whitehead AS, Yunis EJ, Colten HR: Polymorphism of the human complement C4 and steroid 21-hydroxylase genes: Restriction fragment length polymorphisms revealing structural deletions, homoduplications and size variants. J Clin Invest 1986;78:650–657.
20 Mauff G, Alper CA, Dawkins R, Doxiadis G, Giles CM, Hauptmann G, Rittner C, Schneider PM: C4 Nomenclature statement. Complement Inflamm 1990;7:261–268.
21 Giles CM: C4: Rodgers and Chido Typing. Complement Inflamm 1990;7:213–217.
22 Schneider PM: C4 DNA RFLP reference typing report. Complement Inflamm 1990;7:218–224.
23 Rittner C, Stradmann-Bellinghausen B: C4 alpha chain reference typing report. Complement Inflamm 1990;7:225–229.
24 Barba G, Braun-Heimer L, Rittner C, Schneider PM: A new PCR-based typing of the Rodgers and Chido antigenic determinants of the fourth component of human complement. Eur J Immunogenet 1994;21:325–339.
25 Schneider PM, Stradmann-Bellinghausen B, Rittner C: Genetic polymorphism of the fourth component of human complement: population study and proposal for a revised nomenclature based on genomic PCR typing of Rodgers and Chido determinants. Eur J Immunogenet 1996;23:335–344.
26 Mauff G, Suzuki K, Tokunaga K, Hauptmann G, Brenden M, Hasbach H: C4 reference typing report; in Tsuji K, Aizawa M, Sasazuki T (eds): HLA. Oxford, Oxford University Press, 1992, vol 1, pp 954–957.
27 Mauff G, Brenden M, Braun-Stilwell M: Relative electrophoretic migration distances for the classification of C4 allotypes. Complement Inflamm 1990c;7:277–281.
28 Mancini G, Carbonara AO, Heremans JF: Immunochemical quantitation of antigen by single radial immunodiffusion. Immunochemistry 1965;2:235.
29 Holme E, Cross SJ, Veitch J, O'Neill GJ, Whaley K: Quantitation of human C4A and C4B in serum and plasma by enzyme-linked immunoabsorbent assay. Immunogenetics 1988;27:295–297.
30 Moulds JM, Arnett FC, Hamilton RG: A novel immunoassay for the quantitation of human C4 gene products. Complement Inflamm 1990;7:95–101.
31 Belt KT, Caroll MC, Porter RR: The structural basis of the multiple forms of human complement component C4. Cell 1984;36:907–914.
32 Kennedy LJ, Poulton KV, Thomson W, Williams F, Middleton D, Howell WM, Tarassi K, Papasteriades C, Albert E, Fleischauer K, Chandanayingyong D, Tiercy JM, Juji T, Tokunaga K, Ollier WER: HLA class I DNA typing using sequence specific oligonucleoride probes (SSOP); in Charron D (ed): Genetic Diversity of HLA, Functional and Medical Implications. Paris, EDK, 1997, pp 216–225.
33 Kimura A, Sasazuki T: Eleventh International Histocompatibility Workshop reference protocol for the HLA DNA-typing technique; in Tsuji K, Aizawa M, Sasazuki T (eds): HLA. Oxford, Oxford University Press, 1991.
34 Olerup O, Zetterquist H: HLA-DR typing by PCR amplification with sequence-specific primers (PCR-SSP) in 2 hours: an alternative to serological DR typing in clinical practice including donor-recipient matching in cadaveric transplantations. Tissue Antigens 1992;29:225–235.
35 Mauff G: Genetic polymorphism of complement components and other plasma proteins; in Mayr W (ed): Advances in Forensic Haemogenetics. Heidelberg, Springer, 1988, vol 2, pp 133–143.
36 Mauff G, Bender K, Giles CM, Goldmann S, Opferkuch W, Wachauf B: Human C4 polymorphism: Pedigree analysis of qualitative, quantitative, and functional parameters as a basis for phenotype interpretations. Hum Genet 1984;65: 362–372.
37 Geserick G, Otremba P, Schröder H, Stradmann-Bellinghausen B, Schneider PM: Reference typing report for complement factor B. Exp Clin Immunogenet 1998;15:261–263.
38 Weg-Remers S, Brenden M, Schwarz E, Witzel K, Schneider PM, Guerra LK, Rehfeldt IR, Lima MT, Hartmann D, Petzl-Erler ML, de Messias IJT, Mauff G: Major histocompatibility complex (MHC) class III genetics in two Amerindian tribes from southern Brazil: The Kaingang and the Guarani. Hum Genet 1997;100:548–556.

Experimental and Clinical Immunogenetics

Exp Clin Immunogenet 1998;15:261–263

Reference Typing Report for Complement Factor B

G. Geserick[a]
P. Otremba[a]
H. Schröder[a]
B. Stradmann-Bellinghausen[b]
P.M. Schneider[b]

Institute of Legal Medicine,
[a] Humboldt University, Berlin, and
[b] Johannes Gutenberg University, Mainz, Germany

Key Words
Complement
Factor B
Polymorphism
Nomenclature
Electrophoresis
PCR-RFLP

Abstract
Factor B (BF) reference typing was carried out on the occasion of the VIIth Complement Genetics Workshop in Mainz, May 1998. Two different sets of samples were analysed by agarose electrophoresis and/or isoelectric focusing at the protein level, and by PCR-RFLP analysis at the DNA level. These results confirmed the reliability of the standard agarose electrophoresis technique for the identification of the major BF alleles as well as for the identification of cathodic and anodic variants. However, the exact alphanumeric designation of individual variants relative to the reference distance between alleles S and F1 turned out to be more difficult. Using PCR-RFLP analysis, the common alleles F and S as well as the FA and FB subtypes in 6 samples containing an F allele were all assigned correctly. However, the variants F1 and S07 were not detected by this method, as they could not be distinguished from the accompanying S allele. Therefore, a combined application of all three typing methods is recommended for a reliable identification of factor B alleles, variants and FA/FB subtypes.

Introduction

Factor B (BF) reference typing was carried out on the occasion of the VIIth Complement Genetics Workshop in Mainz, May 1998. Two different sets of samples were analysed by agarose electrophoresis and/or isoelectric focusing at the protein level, and by PCR-RFLP analysis at the DNA level. The following seven laboratories participated in the exercise: A. Arnaiz-Villena, Madrid, Spain; M. Brai, Palermo, Italy; M. Cuccia, Pavia, Italy;

KARGER
Fax + 41 61 306 12 34
E-Mail karger@karger.ch
www.karger.com

0254–9670/98/0154–0261$17.50/0

Accessible online at:
http://BioMedNet.com/karger

Prof. Dr. med. Gunther Geserick
Institute of Legal Medicine, Medical Faculty (Charité)
Humboldt University, Hannoversche Strasse 6
D–10115 Berlin (Germany)
Tel. +49 30 2093 7311, Fax +49 30 2093 7546

Table 1. PCR/RFLP typing of factor B allotypes S, FA, and FB [5]

BF PCR allotype	Restriction enzyme	Codon 7 residue	PCR restriction fragments
F	*Msp*I (–)	Trp/Gln	252 bp
S	*Msp*I (+)	Arg	132/120 bp
FB	*Bsl*I (–)	Trp	119/91/42 bp
FA	*Bsl*I (+)	Gln	119/72/42/19 bp
S[a]	*Bsl*I (+)	Arg	119/72/42/19 bp

[a] The 72 bp *Bsl*I fragment is also present in the case of the BF*S allele.

G. Geserick, Berlin, Germany; M. Lokki, Helsinki, Finland; P. Santos, Coimbra, Portugal; L. Truedsson, Lund, Sweden.

Protein Allotyping

Using high-voltage agarose gel electrophoresis (HVAGE) and immunofixation, 19 human plasma samples were analysed by 5 laboratories (Berlin, Helsinki, Lund, Palermo, Pavia). These samples included the common phenotypes F, FS, and S, as well as the variants F155 (in the phenotype F155S), F1 (in F1F), F065 (in F065S), and S07 (in SS07). The typing technology and nomenclature were used as published previously [1–3].

The common phenotypes were all assigned correctly. All variants were detected as well. The alphanumeric designation of these alleles was most consistently achieved for the cathodic variant F1 and the anodic variant S07, except for 1 assignment of S10 for a S07 variant. Minor differences were apparent for the designation of the anodic variant F065, which was identified once as F08, and once as F10. A major difference was observed regarding variant F155, which was designated identically in only two laboratories. The other 4 laboratories assigned designations from F185 to F120.

These results confirmed the reliability of the standard agarose electrophoresis technique for the identification of the major BF alleles as well as for the identification of cathodic and anodic variants. However, the exact alphanumeric designation of individual variants relative to the reference distance between alleles S and F1 turned out to be more difficult. This may in part be the result of an insufficient electrophoretic separation of these alleles, as well as of problems of exact measurement of distances between the protein bands.

Isoelectric Focusing and PCR Typing

Using polyacrylamide gel isoelectric focusing (PAGIF), the BF*F subtypes FA and FB can be identified [2–4]. These subtypes as well as the major alleles F and S can also be distinguished directly at the genomic DNA level using PCR followed by restriction fragment analysis of codon 7 with the enzymes *Msp*I (for F/S typing) and *Bsl*I (for FA/FB typing), as summarized in table 1 [5, 6].

For this part of the exercise, the 11 samples from the C4 reference typing [7] that were available both as plasma and DNA samples were subjected to agarose gel electrophoresis and/or PCR typing in 5 participating laboratories (Berlin, Coimbra, Helsinki, Lund, Madrid). These included the common alleles F and S as well as the variants F1 and S07 in various phenotypic combinations. The common alleles F and S as well as the FA and FB subtypes in 6 samples containing an F allele were all assigned correctly. Using PCR, however, variants F1 and S07 could not be detected by this method, as they could not be distinguished from the accompanying S allele. This has also been noted by Jahn et al. [5], who observed two different F1 variants which were typed either as S or as FB by PCR-RFLP analysis. The authors speculate that the F1 variant carrying the S-like codon 7 exhibits further heterogeneity due to additional amino acid exchanges which change the electrophoretic mobility from S to F1. However, the genetic basis of both the F1 and the S07 variants has not been identified yet.

Conclusions

Due to the complexity of the BF polymorphism both at the DNA and the protein levels, a combined application of all three typing methods – HVAGE, PAGIF and PCR-RFLP – is still required for a reliable identification of factor B alleles, variants and FA/FB subtypes.

References

1 Mauff G, Hauptmann G, Hitzeroth HW, Gauchel F, Scherz R: The nomenclature of properdin factor B allotypes. Z Immunitätsforsch 1978; 154:115–120.

2 Geserick G, Patzelt D: Factor B (BF) subtyping by isoelectric focusing: Methods, nomenclature, genetics and forensic application. Electrophoresis 1988;9:418–421.

3 Geserick G, Abbal M, Brenden M, Braun-Stilwell M, Mauff G, Schröder H, Siemens I: Factor B reference typing report. Complement Inflamm 1990;7:183–189.

4 Geserick G, Abbal M, Mauff G, Siemens I: Factor B (BF) nomenclature statement. Complement Inflamm 1990;7:255–260.

5 Jahn I, Mejia JE, Thomas M, Darke C, Schröder H, Geserick G, Hauptmann G: Genomic analysis of the F subtypes of human complement factor B. Eur J Immunogenet 1994:21: 415–423.

6 Davrinche C, Abbal M, Campbell RD: Molecular characterization of human complement factor B subtypes. Immunogenetics 1990;32: 309–312.

7 Mauff G, Luther B, Schneider PM, Rittner C, Stradmann-Bellinghausen B, Dawkins R, Moulds JM: Reference typing report for complement component C4. Exp Clin Immunogenet 1998;15:249–260.

Experimental and Clinical
Immunogenetics

Exp Clin Immunogenet 1998;15:264–267

Received: November 4, 1998
Accepted: November 6, 1998

C. Rittner[a]
D. Bellavia[b]
G. Geserick[c]
A. Frank[a]
B. Stradmann-Bellinghausen[a]

Reference Typing Report for Complement Component C3

[a] Institute of Legal Medicine, Johannes Gutenberg University, Mainz, Germany,
[b] Istituto di Patologia generale, University of Palermo, Italy,
[c] Institute of Legal Medicine, Humboldt University, Berlin, Germany

Key Words
C3 polymorphism
High-voltage gel electrophoresis
Molecular basis of variants

Abstract
A comparison of five C3 variant samples has been performed by conventional high-voltage gel electrophoresis in three laboratories (Palermo, Berlin and Mainz). Local designation was shown within SD = ±0.75 mm migration distance in the Mainz laboratory. Methodological modifications by laboratories were not accounted for (cooling temperature, relative mobilities between runs). In parallel, all reference samples were also sequenced after exon-specific amplification. As a result, two variants with identical final designations and two variants with different mobilities were shown to conform at the molecular basis exhibiting an amino acid exchange that causes the corresponding change in relative mobility as compared to normal C3F and C3S.

Introduction

The history of C3 variant typing has now completed its third decade [see Alper, 1, this issue]. Nevertheless, the present-day level of detection is still high-voltage agarose electrophoresis, as originally described [2]. In our report of C3 typing during the VIth Complement Genetics Workshop, Mainz, 1989 [3] we had expressed our hope that C3 variant designation would soon be possible at the molecular level by DNA sequencing. Meanwhile, the molecular basis of the electrophoretic variation between C3S and C3F allotypes could be traced to a single C to G transversion at nucleotide 364, in exon 3, leading to the substitution of an arginine residue (positively charged) for a glycine residue (neutral) in C3F [4]. From the same laboratory [6] and another group [5], the genomic organization of human C3 was reported. However, thereafter, only a single report was published on the genomic basis of a rare C3 variant [7].

KARGER
Fax + 41 61 306 12 34
E-Mail karger@karger.ch
www.karger.com

0254–9670/98/0154–0264$17.50/0

Accessible online at:
http://BioMedNet.com/karger

Prof. Dr. Ch. Rittner
Institut für Rechtsmedizin
Johannes Gutenberg-Universität, Am Pulverturm 3
D–55131 Mainz (Germany)
Tel. +49 6131 177 387, Fax +49 6131 393 183

Therefore, a considerable amount of sequencing work still remains to be done to transform the arbitrary electrophoretic approach to C3 variant designation into a molecular map of presumably single or multiple amino acid substitutions leading to those largely observed minute mobility changes in electrophoretic migration which nevertheless were investigated by several authors in the past [8–10]. In this communication and in a forthcoming publication [Frank et al., in preparation], it will be shown that migration differences can be attributed to single amino acid differences at the molecular level (F07 and S045). In contrast, seemingly identical C3 variant allotypes (S035) are so far indistinguishable with regard to their exon structure [11].

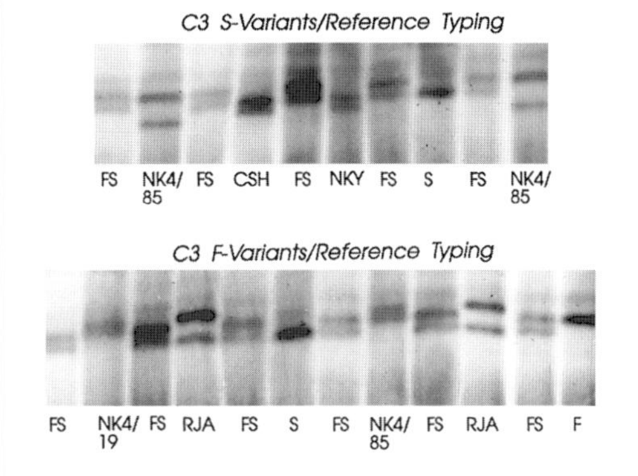

Fig. 1. Electrophoretic comparison of reference samples by the Mainz laboratory.

Material and Methods

Five freshly drawn C3 variant sera from selected individuals were safely shipped on dry ice from Mainz to two reference typing laboratories in Palermo/Italy and Berlin/Germany. The selection was made on the basis of preliminary designations of the Mainz laboratory. Two samples each – NK4/19 and RJA and NKY and CSH (table 1) – were chosen for exhibiting either identical (NKY and CSH) or very similar migration (NK4/19 and RJA). In addition, a different sample (NK4/85) was included. The reference typing was aimed at determining C3 variant migration compared to the standard C3S–F distance [8, 9] in multiple runs as an interlaboratory comparison. No standard protocol of buffer, cooling and other electrophoretic conditions was agreed upon.

Results

A routine separation of all reference samples is shown in figure 1. The results of repeated runs, ranging from a single run to six different electrophoretic separations, were reported by the participating laboratories and finally collected by the reference laboratory in Mainz (table 1). Laboratories were also free to select their own method of measuring migration distances: all three laboratories made overhead projections on paper pinned at a wall. In addition, the Berlin laboratory performed measurements on PC-scanned enlargements of the gel plates. A summary of the reference typing results is given in table 1.

The data in Palermo were obtained by four consecutive measurements after overhead projection of a single electrophoretic run. In Berlin, six different electrophoretic runs were measured by five different individual workers. The Mainz results were obtained by one of the authors (A.F.) in five different runs and evaluated by measurements on overhead projections of each gel.

As can be seen in table 1, there is an overall good agreement among the three laboratories although different approaches to C3 allotyping have been used. In the Mainz laboratory, the mean standard deviation between different measurements was calculated with SD = ±0.75 mm.

Table 1. C3 variant typing in conventional electrophoresis in three reference typing laboratories (Palermo, Berlin and Mainz) in comparison with direct DNA sequencing after exon-specific amplification [Frank et al., 11, and in prep.]

Code	Palermo	Berlin	Mainz	Final designation	cDNA position
NK4/19	F08	F07	F068	F07	not yet determined
RJA	F075	F07	F073	F07	3460 = C/T
NKY	S04	S035	S034	S035	4915 = A/C
CSH	S04	S035	S034	S035	4915 = A/C
NK4/85	S045	S05	S047	S045	2729 = C/G

The molecular substitutions indicated in the right column are taken from Frank et al. [11] as part of molecular heterogeneity detected in exons and their flanking regions as far as amino acid replacements thus emerge. As far as completed, C3 variant allotype F07 in sample RJA can be distinguished from basic C3S sequence by a C to T transition in exon 27 of RJA (in addition to a silent mutation in cDNA position 4956). In contrast, C3 allotype samples NKY and CSH – both designated 'S035' by electrophoretic comparison – share the same substitution at cDNA position 4915 as previously found in a S025 allotype [7]. Similarly, the C to T exchange in sample NK4/85 leads to a substitution of a proline (neutral) for arginine (positively charged, and therefore migrating more slowly than normal C3S allotype).

Discussion and Call for Reference Service

After 30 years of C3 variant typing, the dawn of a molecular genetic interpretation of this abundant polymorphism has come. Many drawbacks of protein investigation such as rapid breakdown of C3, need for repeated bleedings, standardization of electrophoretic method, etc., could thereby be avoided. Still, for the time being, high-voltage electrophoresis will remain a reliable screening method for the selection of C3 allotypes.

The reference laboratory for C3 polymorphism at the Mainz University, still in operation, can add to the published list of reference allotypes sample NK4/85 as a new probe for 'S045' allotype. In addition, a DNA register will be established for sequencing data. Scientists from all over the world are invited to serve the register with their published or unpublished data stating whether access should be given or not. If genomic DNA is received from the authors, a DNA bank could also be opened for reference purposes.

References

1 Alper CA: A history of complement genetics. Exp Clin Immunogenet 1998;15:203–212.
2 Alper CA, Propp RP: Genetic polymorphism of the third component of human complement (C′3). J Clin Invest 1968;47:2181–2191.
3 Rittner C, Stradmann-Bellinghausen B: C3 reference typing report and nomenclature revision. Compl Inflamm 1990;7:230–233.
4 Botto M, Fong KY, So AK, Koch C, Walport MJ: Molecular basis of polymorphisms of human complement component C3. J Exp Med 1990;172:1011–1017.
5 Barnum SR, Amiguet P, Amiguet-Barras F, Fey GH, Tack BF: Complete intron/exon organization of DNA encoding the alpha chain of human C3. J Biol Chem 1989;264: 8471–8474.
6 Fong KY, Botto M, Walport MJ, So AK: Genomic organization of human complement component C3. Genomics 1990;7:579.
7 Höhler T, Botto M, Rittner C, Schneider PM, Meyer zum Büschenfelde KH: Complement component C3: Molecular basis of the C3 S025 variant and evidence for molecular heterogeneity of other variants. Hum Genet 1995;96:539–541.
8 Rittner C, Rittner B: Qualitative and quantitative comparison of C3 variant sera during the Bonn Workshop. Vox Sang 1973;25:21–24.
9 Rittner C, Rittner B: Report 1973/1974 of the Reference Laboratory for the Polymorphism of the Third Component (C3) of the Human Complement System. Vox Sang 1974;27:464–472.
10 Geserick G, Mukaida M, Schröder H: Beobachtungen eines seltenen Phänotyps im C3-System (F065F045) bei einem Paternitätsfall. Nachweis des Erbganges; in Bauer G (ed): Gerichtsmedizin – Festschrift für Wilhelm Holczabeck. Vienna, Deuticke, 1988.
11 Frank A, Stradmann-Bellinghausen B, Schneider PM, Rittner C, Höhler T: Molecular basis of several rare variants and genomic organisation of the human C3 gene. Mol Immunol 1998;35:405.

Experimental and Clinical Immunogenetics

Exp Clin Immunogenet 1998;15:268–285

Received: September 30, 1998
Accepted: October 1, 1998

R. Würzner[a]
K. Witzel-Schlömp[b]
K. Tokunaga[c]
B.A. Fernie[d]
M.J. Hobart[e]
A. Orren[f]

Reference Typing Report for Complement Components C6, C7 and C9 Including Mutations Leading to Deficiencies

[a] Institute of Hygiene, Leopold Franzens University, Innsbruck, Austria;
[b] Institute of Legal Medicine, Johannes Gutenberg University, Mainz, Germany;
[c] Department of Human Genetics, University of Tokyo, Japan;
[d] Centre for Veterinary Science, University of Cambridge, UK;
[e] Department of Biological Sciences, De Montfort University, Leicester, UK;
[f] Department of Microbiology, National University of Ireland, Galway, Ireland

Key Words

Complement · Terminal · Proteins · Genes · Genetics · Allotypes · Polymorphisms · Deficiencies

Abstract

The results of the present (VIIth Complement Genetics Workshop and Conference, Mainz, May 1998) and past reference typing workshops for the terminal complement components C6, C7 and C9 are compiled and discussed both on the protein level and on the DNA level. This report also focusses on the molecular bases of expressed and silent polymorphisms and reviews the molecular bases of subtotal and complete deficiencies of these proteins and their associations with protein and DNA markers. The results of the protein typing for C6 are published in the following paper of this issue.

C6/C7/C9 Workshop

The terminal complement components C6, C7 and C9 are single-chain serum proteins [1] which interact with each other to represent a functional unit [1], and are also biochemically [2] and structurally [3, 4] very similar. Furthermore, they are coded by closely linked genes [5–8] in proximity on chromosome 5p13 [9–13]. All genes are also strongly structurally related [14, 15] and likely derived from one common ancestor [16], which was suggested for C6 and C7 more than 20 years ago [17].

Over recent years the genes of these terminal complement proteins have been studied in detail [12–15, 18]. Knowledge of the gene

KARGER

Fax + 41 61 306 12 34
E-Mail karger@karger.ch
www.karger.com

0254–9670/98/0154–0268$17.50/0

Accessible online at:
http://BioMedNet.com/karger

Reinhard Würzner, MD, PhD
Institute of Hygiene, University of Innsbruck
Fritz-Pregl-Strasse 3, A–6020 Innsbruck (Austria)
Tel. +43 512 507 3426, Fax +43 512 507 2870
E-Mail reinhard.wuerzner@uibk.ac.at

Table 1. Reference typing laboratories for C6 and C7

	C6	C7
Main reference typing laboratory	Geserick, Berlin	Würzner, Innsbruck
Reference samples also available from	Würzner, Innsbruck	Orren, Galway
	Schneider, Mainz	Schneider, Mainz

structure has enabled considerable progress in defining genetic defects responsible for deficiencies of these proteins (C6D and C7D), including apparently total deficiency of C6 (C6Q0), and subtotal deficiencies (C6SD and C7SD). The C6 and C7 but not C9 proteins have been recognized as being polymorphic for some time [5, 19, 20]. The study of the C6 and C7 genes in a number of different populations has revealed that the genes themselves carry both the sequence changes responsible for the protein polymorphisms, and other neutral DNA sequence polymorphisms. These DNA marker polymorphisms are used to determine the C6/C7 DNA marker haplotypes. Certain marker haplotypes are strongly associated with particular C6 or C7 defects and are extremely useful in aiding the study of heterogeneity, epidemiology, provenance and age of these deficiencies [21–23].

The C6/C7/C9 report is divided into seven sections:

C6 protein typing, where all submitted samples were compared with previous reference samples using the elegant direct immunofixation technique, discussing mismatches and accepting new designations for rare C6 allotypes, as the phenotypes need a name irrespective of the fact that a final nomenclature should be introduced once the molecular bases of the allotypes are known. These (serological) results are published in the following paper of this issue.

C7 protein typing, reviewing published data, particularly in respect to the application of the C7 M/N polymorphism. The use of the allospecific monoclonal antibody (MAb) WU 4–15 has shown that the C7 protein in Caucasians is not phenotypically almost monomorphic. Data will also be presented supporting the possible existence of duplicated C7 genes.

C6 and C7 deficiencies and protein typing, revealing the use of polymorphic markers for tracing a deficiency gene of the same or that of a linked protein.

C6 and C7 DNA typing and *Molecular bases of C6 and C7 deficiencies and DNA typing,* reviewing very recently published and unpublished data (i) on the molecular bases of DNA markers and their use for tracing deficiency genes and (ii) on the molecular defects leading to C6 and C7 deficiencies themselves.

C9 DNA typing and *Molecular bases of C9 deficiencies and DNA typing,* presenting very recently published and as yet unpublished data on C9 polymorphisms and deficiencies. At the phenotypic level, however, C9 remains invariant, as no allotypes have been found in all major and a few minor populations investigated. Therefore, no C9 protein typing data are available and hence no report.

For the polymorphic C6 and C7 proteins all available reference samples were collected, retested and stored at three different locations within Europe. One of these laboratories functions as Main Reference Typing Laboratory (table 1).

Table 2. C7 IEF alleles in Caucasians (CAU) and Mongoloids (MON)

	CAU	MON[1]	Comment	Selected references for CAU/JAP/CHI/KOR
C7*1	0.99	0.85	Very common	5 / 31 / 32 / 33
C7*2	<0.01	0.09	Rare/common	5 / 31 / 32 / 33
C7*3	<0.01	0.03	Rare, hypomorphic	5 / 6 / 34 / 33
C7*4	ND	0.04	Rare	5 / 6 / 34 / 33
C7*5[2]			Identical to C7*3	– / 35, 36 / – / –
C7*6			Very rare	– / – / 34 / –
C7*7			Very rare	– / 36 / – / –
C7*8			Very rare	– / 37 / – / –
C7*9[2]			Identical to C7*N	30 / 28 / 38 / –
C7*10			Very rare	Cape Coloureds: 27
C7*R			Very rare, not necessarily different from others mentioned above in Cape Coloureds and Chinese	27, 33

[1] Mean allele frequencies calculated from ten studies with samples from Japanese (JAP), Chinese (CHI) and Koreans (KOR); the mean allele frequency for each population did not differ more than 0.01 from the combined frequency of Mongoloids.

[2] Alleles C7*5 and C7*9 do no longer exist.

As for the other complement proteins, detailed protocols for protein and DNA typing procedures have been recently published elsewhere [24, 25].

C7 Protein Typing

C7 protein typing by isoelectric focusing (IEF) has been extensively studied in Caucasians and Mongoloids (Japanese, Chinese and Koreans), but was also performed using samples from Hindus and Sikhs [26], Cape Coloureds [27], South African Blacks [28], and South American Cayapa Indians [29], by means of polyacrylamide gel IEF, followed by haemolytic overlay or immunoblotting. In Caucasians only one common allele (C7*1) with a gene frequency of 0.99 has been described [5, 17], whereas in the Far East three additional common C7 alleles (frequencies of 0.03–0.09) have been reported, as reviewed [30], as well as a few very rare alleles (table 2). The typical C7 IEF band patterns are shown in figure 1.

Washio et al. [36] demonstrated that C7*5, discovered in Japanese by Nishimukai and Tamaki [35] using neuraminidase-treated samples, corresponds to the C7*3 allele of Caucasians.

In an ELISA based on an allospecific anti-C7 MAb about 7% of the samples did not react despite the presence of C7 in the serum suggesting the existence of a new allele, C7*9, whose product is not detected by the MAb [30]. However, with the help of the C7 IEF-polymorphic Japanese sera it was later shown that this allele corresponds to the C7*N allele of the novel electrically neutral C7 M/N polymorphism [28], discussed below.

The C7*10 allele is difficult to detect because of a complete band-interval cathodal charge shift of C7 10 when compared to C7 1 [27].

The novel C7 M/N polymorphism, which is not based on charge differences but is determined by the reaction pattern of an allospecific MAb in an ELISA [28], has been successfully used to trace the source of C7 after liver transplantation [39, 40] showing that the liver is not, as for C6 [41], the almost exclusive site of synthesis. It has also been widely used in terminal complement deficiency studies (see below). Sensitive and specific C7 M/N typing was also used to show that the bone marrow markedly contributes to the circulating C7 level [40] and that the C7 released by PMNs is, at least in vitro, not taken up from the serum but presumably synthesized by a bone marrow progenitor [42].

At the previous Complement Genetics Workshop (1989) some samples presented with complex C7 IEF patterns and it was speculated that these were from subjects with duplicated C7 genes [43]. When one of these sera was analysed by IEF, press-blotting and detection by the allospecific MAb WU 4–15 that recognizes C7 M, this individual was typed C7 2; after application of biotinylated polyclonal anti-C7 IgG followed by ^{125}I-labelled streptavidin and radioautography, a complex pattern was seen and the bands which were not detected by WU 4–15 appeared to be the gene products of C7*1 and C7*3 [44]. This supports the theory of the presence of duplicated genes in some individuals as at least three C7 gene products appear to be present in this individual: C7 2/C7 M, C7 1/C7 N and C7 3/C7 N.

In contrast to C7 IEF allele frequencies, those for C7*M (and thus C7*N) are very similar for Caucasians and Mongoloids, ranging from 0.775 to 0.82 [28, 38], but different for Blacks from Ecuador and South Africa (0.88 and 0.95, respectively) or for Ecuadorian Cayapa Indians (0.64) as reviewed [45].

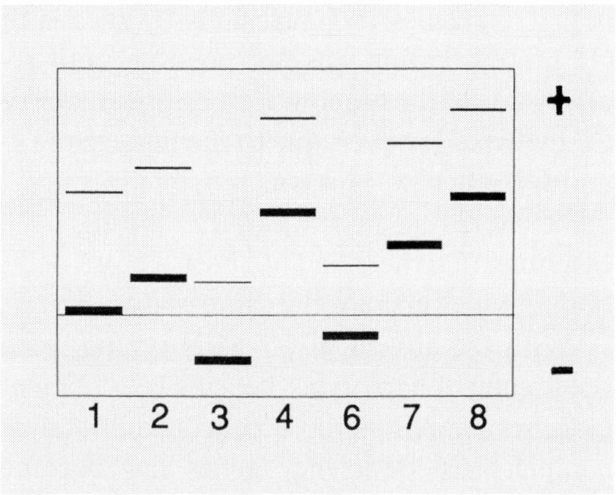

Fig. 1. Schematic illustration and nomenclature of the C7 IEF allotypes [modified from 25]. As for C6, C7 IEF allotypes are characterized by a major and several minor bands (of which the nearest one towards the anode is shown). The numerical nomenclature only relates to the position of the major bands, numbered sequentially according to their discovery. C7 10 shows almost the same band pattern as C7 1 but the most anodal (minor) band is missing and an extra (minor) cathodal band is seen. Thus, the pattern shows a complete band-interval shift towards the cathode which can only be seen when run beside C7 1 samples.

By comparing C7 concentration and haemolytic function of sera of different allotypes, not only C7*3, but also C7*N appeared to be hypomorphic [46]. However, no significant association of C7 alleles to disease has been found [47].

C6 and C7 Deficiencies and Protein Typing

C6 protein typing by IEF has been successfully used to trace haplotypes bearing C6 deficiency genes in families, identifying or excluding homozygous subjects, carriers or unaffected siblings [48]. In contrast, tracing of C7 deficiency genes in Caucasians by means of C7 protein typing was not possible until recently due to the monomorphic appearance of C7 by IEF. However, due to the linkage of C6 and C7 genes [5, 6] it was possible to trace a defective C7 gene via C6 IEF typing [49], assuming that there had not been a cross-over, but not vice versa for the same reason.

With the advent of C7 M/N typing, both the tracing of haplotypes bearing C7 deficiency genes as well as those bearing subtotal or complete C6 deficiency genes has become possible [50]. Furthermore, the method is even sensitive enough to enable the detection of very small amounts of abnormal C7 molecules in four members of the third-generation descendants of a combined subtotal C6/C7-deficient subject, showing that this defective gene is not silent in deficiency gene carriers but expressed [50], whereas no aberrant bands of the abnormal C6 could be identified in these heterozygous subjects by IEF [51, 52]. In this respect C7 M/N typing is even more informative than DNA typing (discussed below) which will assess the presence but not necessarily the functional status of a defective gene.

C7 M/N typing has also proven useful in determining the cause of phenotypic complete C7 deficiency in a Russian subtotal C7D subject with anomalous response to transfusion therapy. The source of C7 appearing after transfusion was ascribed to the patient himself, and not to the transfused material [53, 54], demonstrating his ability to secrete low amounts of the C7 protein.

Both C6 IEF and C7 M/N typing may be used to trace the recently discovered mutations leading to C9 deficiency (see below) but, considering the multiple (mostly non-expressed markers) in that area and the possibility of identifying the mutations themselves (see below), DNA typing appears superior to protein typing in this respect.

C6 and C7 DNA Typing

A rapidly increasing number of polymorphic markers for linked C6 and C7 loci have been described and mapped (table 3). DNA markers have uses:

(a) As normal genetic markers for population studies etc.

(b) To determine the type of protein which would be made if the defective genes of deficient individuals were expressed.

Taken together, a suitable selection of the markers provides a very discriminating tool (a haplotype) for identifying a segment of the chromosome with a possible common inheritance. In this regard, it is noteworthy both that most of the balanced polymorphic markers are present in most human population groups and that allelic association (linkage disequilibrium) is generally rather weak, so that most populations undoubtedly contain tens of different haplotypes. In contrast, in all cases where several examples of a specific gene defect have been investigated, it has usually been found to be strongly associated with one haplotype, and sometimes also with haplotypes which vary at only one or two points from the consensus. Thus in addition to raw marker data, haplotype analysis permits:

(c) the positive identification of inheritance patterns of traits within families.

(d) The identification of probable gene defects in cases of deficiency (though specific confirmatory investigation must be undertaken).

(e) A more advanced tool for population studies, including biological anthropology.

(f) An advanced tool for the detailed description of the context of 'rare' phenotypic alleles.

A shorthand has been introduced for the polymorphic C6 and C7 sites, reflecting the genomic order, and for the time being (until

Table 3. Alleged DNA markers in the C6/C7 region

Gene	Phenotype	Amino acid	Change	Exon	Intron	Enzyme	Frequency	References
C6	A/B	E98A	413A/C	3		*Dde I*	0.35	55, 56
C6			CCGG/CTGG		3	*Msp I*	0.35	57–59
C6		C518C		10		*Bsm I*	Pacific	60
C6			Combindel		10		0.05	61
C6		D544G		11		*Aci I*		60
C6		D544D		11		*Acc I*	0.22	60
C6		Q546H		11		*Bsr I*	0.4	60
C6		R575E		11		*Mnl I*	0.4	60
C6		E630G		12		*Scr FI*		60
C6		R680W		13		*Mae II*	0.1	60
C6					16?	*Taq I*	0.4	7, 62
C7			A/T		15–37			63
C7					15	*Taq I* (225)	0.2	21, 62
C7					13	*Taq I* (233)	0.33	62
C7		T576S	1792A/T	13		*BsrG I*	0.12	23
C7	M/N	T565P	1769A/C	13		*Rsa I*	0.23	28, 62
C7			A/C	12–27			0.17	64
C7			A/C	11+18		Jap. C7 D assoc.		65
C7		S367T	1162G/C	9		*Dde I*	0.37	62, 66, 67
C7			ins T		8+42			63
C7			T/C		7–9			63
C7			T/A		1+55	*Apo I*		63
C7			A/C		1+29			63

The markers are arranged in genome order, with the 3′ C7 markers listed before the 5′ C7 markers. The agreed nomenclature for mutations [68] has been used for the allelic variants, where possible. In all cases, the more common allele in Caucasians is quoted first. cDNA positions are given for coding substitutions, and the consequent amino acid substitutions (mature polypeptide numbering). Intronic markers are numbered (where possible) from the nearest boundary of the intron: positions at the 5′ end of the intron are counted in positive numbers, positions at the 3′ end of the intron are counted in negative numbers from the boundary of the next exon. The enzyme indicated is that which reveals the allelic difference, if an enzyme site is present in either allele. Allele frequencies are quoted for the least common allele in Caucasian (European) populations and are largely based on laboratory personnel: they are approximate at the second significant figure. Markers which are restricted (as far as is known) to distinct population groups are indicated by a short form of the name of that population group: 'Jap. C7 D assoc.' means that the marker was found, so far uniquely, associated with a molecular defect of C7 in a Japanese individual. 'Pacific' means Melanesian Pacific islanders. 'Combindel' means 'combined insertion/deletion'. Numbers in parentheses refer to cDNA probes [66].

further 5′ located markers are discovered) starting with the C6 A/B and C6 MspI polymorphisms, separating C6 and C7 markers by a semicolon, e.g. B+;M being a rather incomplete haplotype (considering the multiple markers in that area) consisting of C6 B, C6 MspI + and C7 M [22, 62].

The molecular basis of the C7 M/N polymorphism is of particular interest as this neutral amino acid substitution is about 40 amino acid residues apart from the epitope of the MAb. Thus, 565-Thr (C7 M) allows access of the MAb to its epitope but its substitution by Pro (C7 N) almost completely inhibits it [28], possibly by disrupting the β sheet structure in that region [P.M. Schneider and R.W., unpubl. data].

Molecular Bases of C6 and C7 Deficiencies and DNA Typing

Individuals with C6D or C7D are usually ascertained because affected individuals have increased susceptibility to neisserial infections, although not all cases give a positive history of these infections [69]. Nevertheless, the ascertainment of C6 and C7 deficiency is markedly affected by the prevalence of meningococcal infections. Tables 4 and 5 summarize the defects in the C6 or C7 genes responsible for C6D or C7D that were known and discussed at the VIIth Complement Genetics Workshop, Mainz, May 1998, including those reported for the first time at that meeting. The tables list defects occurring in independent chromosomes, and therefore do not distinguish as to whether these were studied in individuals, or in families. Ascertainment was either because of meningococcal infections, population screening or, in some cases of subtotal deficiency, through complement investigations because of other medical conditions.

Complete Deficiencies of C6

Reported defects leading to C6 deficiency are summarized in table 4. Three different defects leading to apparently total C6 deficiency have been reported previously. One defect has been reported from Japan, and two (1195delC and 1936delG) in Afro-Americans living in the United States [70, 73]. The same latter two defects are now reported as segregating in the Western Cape, South Africa, as well as occurring in a UK patient of Afro-Caribbean origin [71, 72]. Another defect (879delG) is now reported at this meeting; it has been found, or deduced, in 30 independent chromosomes from Cape Coloured subjects from the Western Cape [71, 72]. This is by far the most prevalent defect yet reported. Why it is segregating in this particular population, and the origin of the defect are not yet known. The Cape Coloureds are descended from the early inhabitants of the Western Cape, as well as people who moved in from Europe, mainly the Netherlands and Britain, from other parts of Africa, and from South-East Asia. C6 deficiency has also been reported from the Netherlands [80], and it was interesting to determine in two Dutch C6D families that three of the four affected chromosomes carried the same 879delG defect that was found in the Cape Coloured C6Q0 patients. However, the DNA marker data show that at least one of the 879delG defects, and very possibly all of them, occur within C6/C7 DNA haplotype(s) different from the common Cape C6Q0 haplotype, indicating a different origin of at least one of the Dutch defects.

Subtotal C6 and Combined C6/C7 Deficiencies

The C6 intron 15 splice donor site defect responsible for subtotal C6 deficiency was the first molecular defect for C6 or C7 to be described [74, 75]. This defect is interesting

Table 4. Molecular defects of the C6 gene leading to C6 deficiency

Common name	Location of C6 defect	Nature of the defect	Number of reported independent affected chromosomes	Predominant geographical areas/affected population (number affected)	Notes	References
C6D[1]	Exon 2	Deletion of one C at position 291 (or 292–294)	1	Japan (1)	Defect produces a frame shift, codons for 42 abnormal amino acids and a premature stop codon	70
C6Q0[2] 879delG	Exon 6	Position 879 is 1st of a run 7 Gs, and arbitrarily ascribed as the deletion site in the run	33 (Including Cape defects deduced because of DNA haplotype data)	Western Cape, SA (30) Netherlands (3)	Premature termination. Marker haplotypes in the Cape indicate a common and ancient origin of the defect; possibly different from that in the Netherlands	71, 72
C6D[1]/C6Q0[2] 1195delC	Exon 7	Deletion of C at position 1195	8 (Including Cape defects deduced because of DNA haplotype data)	Afro-American (2) Western Cape, SA (6)	Production of a premature termination codon	71–73
C6D[1]/C6Q0[2] 1936delG	Exon 12	Deletion of G at nucleotide position 1936	5	Afro-American (4) Western Cape, SA (1)	Frame shift and premature termination codon. The putative polypeptide chain would lack the 3′ one 1/3 of the molecule	70–73
Subtotal C6 deficiency (C6 SD)	5′ Splice donor site of intron 15	T > G preventing normal splicing	1 (Confirmed C6SD without C7SD)	Western Cape, SA	C6 molecule reduced by ~ 14% at 3′ end. Low levels a functionally active molecule produced	74
C6 defect in combined subtotal C6/C7 deficiency	5′ Splice donor site of intron 15, i.e. identical to C6SD above	T > G preventing normal splicing	6 (Confirmed combined C6/C7 SD) 1 (Unconfirmed)	UK(4), Western Cape, SA (1), Russia (1), Germany (1)	C6 molecule as above. Marker haplotypes the same in all confirmed cases, and probably in unconfirmed German case	74, 75
Unknown but investigated			7	Japan (1) Germany (1) UK (2), Ireland (2) Netherlands (1)	All patients have been investigated but defects not yet identified	70–72, 75 (not all are referenced)

The defects are ordered according to the gene location. [1] and [2] refer to C6 deficiency associated with undetectable functional C6, and usually with susceptibility to neisserial infections. This is referred to as C6D or C6Q0 according to terminology used by the authors.

because it has been found both as an isolated defect, and together with subtotal C7 deficiency (subtotal combined C6/C7 deficiency (C6/C7SD)). Although no reason for these two defects to be found together on one chromosome has been determined, the defects coexist in at least six (probably seven), of the eight instances that this intron 15 C6 gene defect has been found. Moreover, although occurring in individuals from widely spaced geographical areas, all chromosomes carrying the combined C6/C7SD defect also carry an identical marker haplotype [75].

Table 5. Molecular defects of the C7 gene leading to C7 deficiency

Common name	Location of C7 defect	Nature of the defect	Number of reported independent affected chromosomes	Predominant geographical areas/affected population (number affected)	Notes	References
C7D	Intron 1/ exon 2 boundary	G > A transition at 3′ acceptor site of intron 1	1	Ireland (1)	G > A affects invariant AG and would cause splice failure	76
Subtotal C7 deficiency	Exon 6	G > A transversion position 659 and substitution Arg by Gln (R198Q)	1	Malta (1)		63, 77
C7 exons 7 and 8 deletion defect	Exons 7 and 8	Deletion of around ~ 6.8 kbp including exons 7 and 8	5	Ireland (5)	Marker haplotypes the same except on one chromosome where 1 C6 marker differs. Both the absence of exons, and splicing abnormality could cause the deficiency	76, 78
C7D	Intron 7	G > A transversion at 5′ splice donor site	1	Russia (1)	Splice failure reading 15 intronic codons before termination	63, 77
C7D	Exon 9	G > C transversion at position 1135 and substitution of Gly by Arg (G357R)	8	Israel/Moroccan Sephardic Jews (8)	Marker haplotypes all the same except on one chromosome where 2 C6 markers differ. The reason for the failure to secrete the abnormal protein not clear	76
Subtotal C7 deficiency	Exon 11	C > A transversion at position 1561 leading to substitution of Arg by Ser at 499 (R449S)	1 (Confirmed exon 11 C7SD defect without C6SD)	Russia	Replacement of Ser by Arg responsible for protein charge difference, but has not been confirmed to be responsible for deficiency. However, this is strongly supported by patient data	75
C7 defect in combined subtotal C6/C7 deficiency	Exon 11	C > A (see above)	6 (Confirmed combined C6/C7 SD) 1 (Unconfirmed)	UK (4), Western Cape, SA (1), Russia (1), Germany (1)	Marker haplotypes the same in all confirmed cases, and probably in unconfirmed case; also see above	75
C7D	Exon 14	1 bp deletion position 1929–1933	1	Russia (1). The patient also had the C7SD defect	Phase change and translation of 10 codons before termination	63, 77
C7D	Exon 14	G > C transversion at position 2044 and substitution of Glu by Gln (E660Q)	1	Western Cape SA/ Cape Coloured (1)		63, 77
C7D	Exon 14	G > A transversion at position 2060 and substitution of Arg by His (R665H)	1	Western Cape/ Cape Coloured (1); the same individual as above		63, 77
C7D	Exon 15	2-bp deletion (2137delTG or 2138delGT or 2139delTG)	2	Japan (2)	The 2-bp deletion results in a frame shift, one different amino acid and a premature termination codon	65
C7D	Exon 16	T > A at nucleotide 2250	2	Japan (2)	A termination codon TGA is generated, leading to truncation	65

Table 5 (continued)

Common name	Location of C7 defect	Nature of the defect	Number of reported independent affected chromosomes	Predominant geographical areas/affected population (number affected)	Notes	References
C7D	Exon 16	Deletion of G at position 2350	1	South African White (1)	Out of phase splice between exons 16 and 17 and premature termination	63, 77
C7D	Intron 16	T > C transversion at 5′ splice donor site of intron 16	1	South African White (1); the same individual as above	Splice failure and reading of 17 intronic codons before termination	63, 77
Unknown but investigated			5	Russia (2), Malta (1) (C7SD), Northern Ireland (2)	All patients have been investigated but defects not yet identified	63, 77 79

The defects are ordered according to the gene location.

Deficiencies of C7

At the present time many more different defects leading to C7 deficiency have been reported (table 5). Six defects, including the one responsible for C7SD in C6/C7SD and as isolated C7D, have been reported previously [65, 75, 76, 78]. At this meeting a further 7 defects were described [63, 77], making a total of 13 different known C7 defects. Most of these appear sporadic and have been only found in one or two independent chromosomes. Nevertheless, C7D can occur with a relatively high frequency in certain populations. A defect at nucleotide position 1135 in exon 9 has been found in eight independent chromosomes in Jews of Moroccan Sephardic descent living in Israel, and an unusual deletion of around 6.8 kbp, including exons 7 and 8, has been found in five independent chromosomes in Ireland [76, 78].

It is not always possible to distinguish genotypic total C7 deficiency from subtotal deficiency. A study of a patient with virtually no C7 in his circulation showed that he carried the same C6/C7SD defects as the other C6/C7SD subjects, as well as another C7 defect [54, 75]. The presence of C5b6 in the circulation led to a consumption of the low amounts of secreted C7. In contrast, patients with the combined deficiency apparently do not have sufficient C6 to allow the production of circulating C5b6, and these subjects have detectable low levels of C7 in the circulation [75]. As far as we know, none of the other C7 defects listed in table 5 occurred together with a C6 defect, and thus any low levels of C7 produced by genes carrying the defects could be masked by circulating C5b6. This is almost certainly true of the Russian brothers with the exon 11 position 1561 C7SD defect that occurred without C6SD [75]. Nevertheless, the subject from Malta reported at this meeting with the exon 6 position 659 G > A transversion, and another as yet unknown C7SD defect, is C6 sufficient and was also shown to have low levels two different C7 allotypes in her circulation, despite the presence of circulating C6 and thus C5b6 [63, 77].

Conclusion

Five different C6 gene defects on 55 independently ascertained chromosomes, and 13 different C7 gene defects on 34 independently ascertained chromosomes have so far been

Table 6. Polymorphic sites in the human complement C9 gene (Codon changes are marked by bold letters)

Position of polymorphism		Changed			Typing method
Exon/intron	cDNA pos.	sequence (5′ → 3′)	amino acid	AA-No.	
Ex 1	17	GCCTGC$^{\mathbf{C}}_{\mathbf{T}}$**GG**AGCT	Arg ↔ Trp	5 (LP)	PCR/RFLP
Int 1	–10 Ex 2	TGTTCT$^{A}_{G}$TTATCT	–	–	Allele-specific PCR
Ex 4	391	CTTT**TC**$^{\mathbf{A}}_{\mathbf{C}}$GATGAG	Ser	108	Allele-specific PCR
Ex 11	1847	TTTTTT$^{T}_{A}$AATTTT	–	–	PCR/RFLP

reported. Tables 4 and 5 also show the position of the defects. The defects occur in a wide range of positions in both the C6 and the C7 genes. It is worth noting that 7 of the 13 different C7 gene defects occur at the 3′ end of the gene in exons 14–16. The most 3′ of the C6 defects is the 5′ splice donor site defect in intron 15 of the C6 gene and it is responsible for coding for a truncated C6SD protein [74]. However, the 3′ C7 gene defects are all associated with what appears to be total C7 deficiency; although, as discussed above, this does not exclude the secretion of low levels of C7. The tables also refer to some C6- and C7-deficient subjects who have been investigated, but either one or both defects have remained elusive. For the majority of these subjects this indicates that the unknown defect is not one of the defects listed in the relevant table. Thus there are many defects that have not yet been determined. Reasons for failure to detect defects when the coding exons are sequenced have been discussed [77]. It was concluded that this is either because the defects are not within the coding exons, or because of PCR failure which can occur with exon deletions (cf. the C7 exons 7 and 8 deletion), or when an unknown polymorphism occurs within the footprint of a primer.

C9 DNA Typing

Despite the monomorphic appearance of the C9 molecule, several polymorphic sites have been detected at the cDNA level by Southern blot analysis, each creating a Taq I-RFLP [81, 82]. The exact position of these sites is not known yet. In the course of C9 deficiency studies (see below) four additional polymorphic sites have been found in the C9 gene using exon-specific PCR and direct sequencing [15, 83]. As expected, none of them changes the amino acid composition of the mature protein (table 6):

A C/T transition was found in exon 1 at cDNA position 17. Thus, the fifth amino acid (aa) of the leader peptide may either be an arginine or a tryptophan. Although these two aa have different properties, C9 seems to be secreted irrespective of the residue present, as several probands having one or the other variant in comparable concentrations have been observed. The C-allele is characterized by a Msp I restriction site (C↓CGG).

An A/G transition is located in intron 1, 10 bp upstream of the boundary to exon 2. It does not change the respective splice site.

An A/C transversion in exon 4 at cDNA position 391 changes the codon for $serine_{108}$ from TCA to TCC.

An A/T exchange was found in the 3′ untranslated region of exon 11 at cDNA position 1847. The A-allele is characterized by a Dra I-recognition site (TTT↓AAA).

Using either PCR/RFLP analysis (Msp I, exon 1 and Dra I, exon 11) or allele-specific PCR (intron 1 and exon 4), each of the polymorphisms can be characterized without sequencing [83]. A large number of genomic DNA samples from three population groups of different geographic origin (54 Europeans, 16 Thais, and 8 South-American Indians [84]) were screened for these four markers. The exon 1-, intron 1-, and exon 11-alleles were all found within each population. Thus, they probably arose from a common ancestor. In contrast, the exon 4 C-variant was observed only once in a European in the course of this study and previously in a Swiss proband with heterozygous C9 deficiency. Therefore, the mutation presumably arose more recently in Europe.

Disregarding the exon 4 site, eight different C9 haplotypes can theoretically be described. Six of them have actually been observed [83], their frequences reflecting those of the single alleles. The haplotypes T/A/A and T/G/A (exon 1/intron 1/exon 11) were missing, possibly because of the low exon 11 A-frequence. The exon 4 C-variant was linked to the most common haplotype C/G/T in both cases. The haplotype T/A/T was observed in one quarter of the European genes analysed, but missing in the other populations.

The data provide strong evidence for several mutation and recombination events in the course of the C9 gene evolution. Nevertheless, strong selection forces prevented point mutations in the coding sequence giving rise to C9 allotypes. Additional polymorphisms, located in one of the long C9 introns not analysed yet (as for the Taq I RFLPs detected by Southern blot [81, 82]) may be detected in subsequent studies.

Molecular Bases of C9 Deficiencies and DNA Typing

C9 deficiency leads to incomplete membrane attack complex formation and may therefore predispose to recurrent neisserial infections [69, 85]. In contrast to the situation in Japan, where C9 deficiency has a very high incidence (0.045–0.104%) [86–89], it is a rare finding in Europe [90, 91]. This may be, in part, due to the different methods used in Japan and Europe [91]: the CH50 at low strength, as routinely done in Japan, favours the detection of C9D, whereas the sucrose-GVB buffer routinely used in Europe may only yield values just outside or even still within the normal range. Interestingly, the use of guinea pig or fowl erythrocytes in the alternative pathway APCH50 allows the detection of C9D, whereas the use of rabbit red blood cells does not [91].

Using exon-specific PCR and direct sequencing of each of the 11 C9 exons [15, 83] the genetic bases for the lack of C9 in the serum of three unrelated European individuals, one of Swiss and two of Irish origin, were identified. Only one of them suffered from two episodes of bacterial meningitis [90]. Five different point mutations were detected altogether (table 7), four of them generating a TGA stop codon in the coding sequence of exons 2, 4, and 9, respectively, and the fifth causing a Cys to Gly codon change in exon 4.

Each of these complete C9-deficient Caucasian subjects was a compound heterozygote, i.e. two different mutations were found, each in heterozygous status: Two stop codons were detected in the C9 genes of the Swiss proband, one is located in exon 2 (aa position 33) and

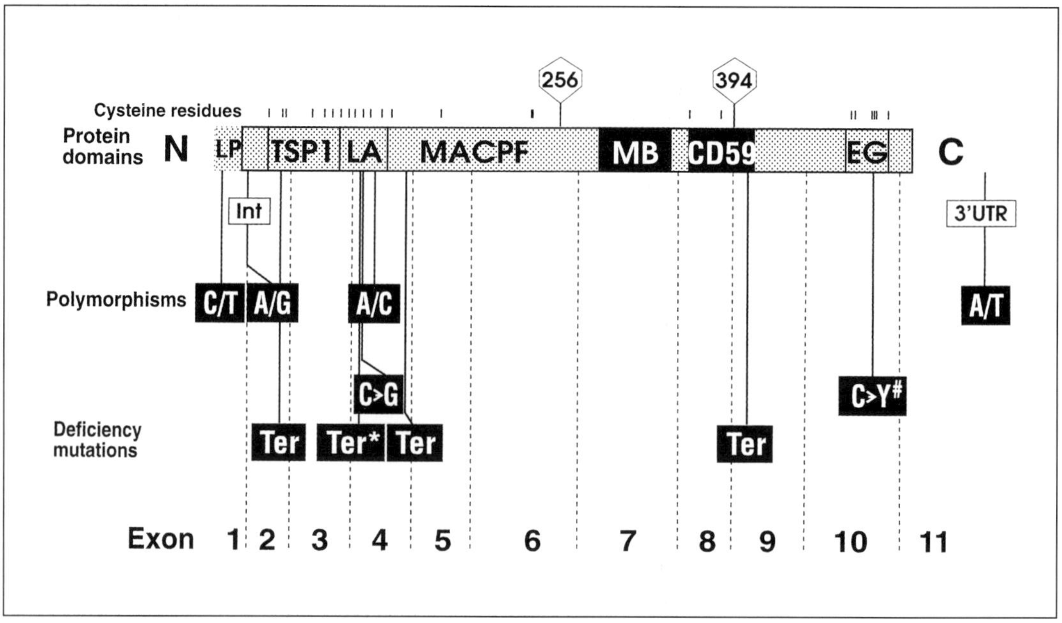

Fig. 2. Structure of the C9 protein [modified from 1] and positions of polymorphisms and mutations causing C9 deficiency. Regions showing significant homology to sequences of other proteins are the thrombospondin type 1 module (TSP1), the low density lipoprotein-receptor class A module (LA), and the epidermal growth factor module (EG). Additional C9 protein domains are the leader peptide (LP) and a region with sequence similarity between the members of the MAC family and perforin (MACPF). The membrane binding (MB) region as well as the amino acids recognized by CD59 (CD59) are located in the MACPF. Glycosylated asparagin residues are represented by hexagons, cysteine residues by vertical lines. Additional abbreviations correspond to introns (Int), 3′ untranslated region (3′ UTR), and termination codon (Ter). For polymorphisms the allelic nucleotides are given, for deficiency mutations not creating a stop codon, the amino acid exchanges are represented in the one letter code. Mutations also found in concurrent studies are marked (* [93, 94], # [93]).

Table 7. Point mutations leading to C9 deficiency

Position of mutation		Change of		AA-No.	Observed with
exon	cDNA pos. [1]	codon	amino acid		
2	166	TG**C** → TG**A**	Cys → Stop	33	Swiss [15, 90], Irish X [91, 92]
4	350	**C**GA → **T**GA	Arg → Stop	95	Irish X [91, 92], Japanese [93, 94]
4	359	**T**GT → **G**GT	Cys → Gly	98	Irish Y [92]
4	464	**C**GA → **T**GA	Arg → Stop	133	Swiss [15, 90]
9	1284	T**C**A → T**G**A	Ser → Stop	406	Irish Y [92]
10	1587	T**G**T → T**A**T	Cys → Tyr	507	Japanese [93]

[1] cDNA position according to the the sequence deposited in the EMBL Data Base, Acc. No. X02176

the other one in exon 4 at aa position 133 [15]. The Irish proband X likewise carrys the exon 2 stop codon and, in addition, he has the TGA stop codon in exon 4 at aa position 95 [92]. In the Irish subject Y, the stop codon in exon 9 (aa position 406) and the cysteine to glycine exchange in exon 4 (aa position 98) were observed [92]. Family studies of two index cases, the Swiss and the Irish Y, revealed that these mutations segregate independently and are thus sufficient to explain the subjects' inherited C9 deficiency.

One of proband Y's mutated gene products still seems to be secreted and even functionally active [92] as demonstrated by ELISA studies, measuring incorporation of C9 molecules into the terminal complement complex (TCC) [95, 96] and haemolytic agarose gel diffusion assay [91, 97]. The hypothetical product of the allele bearing the exon 9 stop codon would comprise 405 aa residues. Thus, it would include important regions, like the membrane-inserting domain and C8/C9 binding epitopes [1] (fig. 2). However, the truncation will probably prevent the correct folding of the protein. Alternatively, the detected C9 molecules may be translation products of proband Y's other allele. In this case, the lack of a cysteine codon will probably also result in a protein of different conformation, as one of the intramolecular disulfide bridges cannot be formed [98].

No C9 could be demonstrated in the serum of the Swiss and the Irish proband X, i.e. their phenotypes are of complete C9 deficiency [92]. In either of these cases, the in-phase stop codons would lead to hypothetical translation products with minimal lengths, respectively, thus lacking functional important domains of the C9 protein (fig. 2).

The observed heterogeneity in the genetic bases for human C9 deficiency in the European population suggests that this deficiency has originated from several independent mutations. Different results were obtained in two concurrent studies from the Far East employing the same technique or PCR followed by single-strand confirmation polymorphisms analysis (SSCP), respectively, and investigating four complete C9-deficient Japanese patients who had suffered from meningococcal meningitis [94] or ten unrelated complete C9 deficient Japanese individuals [93] (table 7). In each individual the same exon 4 stop codon at aa position 95 was found which was also observed in the Irish subject X. All 4 subjects of the former and 8 of the latter study were homozygous, and the remaining 2 were heterozygous for this defect. Thus, one single mutation seems to be the major cause for C9 deficiency in the Japanese population. One of the two different remaining mutations of the two heterozygous Japanese subjects has also been mapped: it is located in exon 10 and changes the $codon_{507}$ from Cys (TGT) to Tyr (TAT). Thus, once more an intramolecular disulfide bond cannot be formed in the respective translation product.

References

1 Plumb ME, Sodetz JM: Proteins of the membrane attack complex; in Volanakis JE, Frank MM (eds): The Human Complement System in Health and Disease. New York, Dekker, 1998, pp 119–148.

2 Podack ER, Kolb WP, Esser AF, Müller-Eberhard HJ: Structural similarities between C6 and C7 of human complement. J Immunol 1979;123:1071–1077.

3 DiScipio RG, Hugli TE: The molecular architecture of human complement component C6. J Biol Chem 1989;264:16197–16206.

4 Reid KB, Day AJ: Structure-function relationships of the complement components. Immunol Today 1989;10:177–180.

5 Hobart MJ, Joysey V, Lachmann PJ: Inherited structural variation and linkage relationships of C7. J Immunogenet 1978;5:157–163.

6 Tokunaga K, Dewald G, Omoto K, Juji T: Family study on the polymorphism of the sixth and seventh components (C6 and C7) of human complement: Linkage and haplotype analyses. Am J Hum Genet 1986;39:414–419.

7 Coto E, Martinez-Naves E, Dominguez O, DiScipio RG, Urra JM, Lopez-Larrea C: DNA polymorphisms and linkage relationship of the human complement component C6, C7 and C9 genes. Immunogenetics 1991;33:184–187.

8 Rogne S, Myklebost O, Olving JH, Kyrkjebo HT, Jonassen R, Olaisen B, Gedde-Dahl T: The human genes for complement component-6 (C6) and component-9 (C9) are closely linked on chromosome 5. J Med Genet 1991;28:587–590.

9 Jeremiah SJ, Abbott CM, Murad Z, Povey S, Thomas HJ, Solomon E, DiScipio RG, Fey GH: The assignment of the genes coding for human complement components C6 and C7 to chromosome 5. Ann Hum Genet 1990;54:141–147.

10 Rogne S, Myklebost O, Stanley K, van Kessel AG: The gene for human complement C9 is on chromosome 5. Genomics 1989;5:149–152.

11 Abbott C, West L, Povey S, Jeremiah S, Murad Z, DiScipio R, Fey G: The gene for human complement component C9 mapped to chromosome 5 by polymerase chain reaction. Genomics 1989;4:606–609.

12 Hobart MJ, Fernie BA, DiScipio RG, Lachmann PJ: A physical map of the C6 and C7 complement component gene region on chromosome–5p13. Hum Mol Genet 1993; 2:1035–1036.

13 Setien F, Alvarez V, Coto E, DiScipio RG, Lopez-Larrea C: A physical map of the human complement component C6, C7 and C9 genes. Immunogenetics 1993;38:341–344.

14 Hobart MJ, Fernie BA, DiScipio RG: Structure of the human C7 gene and comparison with the C6, C8a, C8b and C9 genes. J Immunol 1995; 154:5188–5194.

15 Witzel-Schlömp K, Späth PJ, Hobart MJ, Fernie BA, Rittner C, Kaufmann T, Schneider PM: The human complement C9 gene: Identification of two mutations leading to deficiency and revision of the gene structure. J Immunol 1997; 158:5043–5049.

16 Hobart MJ: Evolution of the terminal complement genes: Ancient and modern. Exp Clin Immunogenet 1998;15:235–243.

17 Hobart MJ, Lachmann PJ: Allotypes of complement components in man. Transplant Rev 1976;32:26–42.

18 Hobart MJ, Fernie BA, DiScipio RG: Structure of the human C6 gene. Biochemistry 1993;32:6198–6205.

19 Hobart MJ, Lachmann PJ, Alper CA: Polymorphism of human C6; in Peters H (eds): Protides of the Biological Fluids. Oxford, Pergamon Press, 1975, p 575–580.

20 Hobart MJ: Phenotypic genetics of complement components. Philos Trans R Soc Lond B 1984;306:325–331.

21 Coto E, Martinez-Naves E, Dominguez O, Lopez-Larrea C: DNA polymorphism of the human complement component C7 gene in familial deficiencies. Hum Genet 1990;85: 251–252.

22 Fernie BA, Orren A, Würzner R, Jones AM, Potter PC, Lachmann PJ, Hobart MJ: Complement component C6 and C7 haplotypes associated with deficiencies of C6. Ann Hum Genet 1995;59:183–195.

23 Fernie BA, Orren A, Schlesinger M, Würzner R, Platonov AE, Cooper RC, Williams YE, Hobart MJ: DNA haplotypes of the complement C6 and C7 genes associated with deficiencies of the seventh component; and a new DNA polymorphism in C7 exon 13. Ann Hum Genet 1997; 61:287–298.

24 Mauff G, Würzner R: Complement genetics; in Herzenberg LA, Weir DM, Herzenberg LA, Blackwell C (eds): Weir's Handbook of Experimental Immunology. Oxford, Blackwell, 1996, vol 2, pp 77.1–77.11.

25 Schneider PM, Rittner C: Complement genetics; in Dodds AW, Sim RB (eds): Complement – A Practical Approach. Oxford, Oxford University Press, 1997, pp 165–198.

26 Corbo RM, Tartaglia M, Scacchi R, Rickards O, Dash S, Sharma SK, Ramdeo IN, Sangatramani TC, Vyas M, Modiano G: A survey of six genetic markers on the populations of Punjab and Rajasthan (India). Gene Geogr 1991;5:113–121.

27 Orren A, Würzner R, Lachmann PJ, Hobart MJ: A novel human complement component C7 phenotype detected in South Africa and proposed designation of the allele as C7*10. Eur J Immunogenet 1994;21:181–187.

28 Würzner R, Hobart MJ, Orren A, Tokunaga K, Nitze R, Götze O, Lachmann PJ: A novel protein polymorphism of human complement C7 detected by a monoclonal antibody. Immunogenetics 1992;35: 398–402.

29 Scacchi R, Corbo RM, Rickards O, De Stefano GF: The Cayapa Indians of Ecuador: A population study of seven protein genetic polymorphisms. Ann Hum Biol 1994;21:67–77.

30 Würzner R, Nitze R, Götze O: C7*9, a new frequent allele detected by an allotype-specific monoclonal antibody. Complement Inflamm 1990;7:290–297.

31 Nakamura S, Ooue O, Abe K: Genetic polymorphism of the seventh component of complement in a Japanese population. Hum Genet 1984;66:279–281.

32 York LJ, Marshall WH, Huang SN: Polymorphism of the seventh complement component, C7, in Chinese. Hum Hered 1986;36:261–262.

33 Park KS, Yanagisawa M, Tokunaga K, Omoto K: Genetic polymorphisms of complement components C6 and C7 in Korean. Jpn J Hum Genet 1988;33:325–331.

34 Zeng Z, Tokunaga K, Omoto K, Du C: Genetic polymorphisms of complement C6 and C7 in two Chinese populations. Jpn J Hum Genet 1986;31:263–271.

35 Nishimukai H, Tamaki Y: Genetic polymorphism of the seventh component of complement: A new variant. Vox Sang 1986;51:60–62.

36 Washio K, Tokunaga K, Omoto K, Misawa S: Human C7 polymorphism: Classification and association analysis with C6. Jpn J Hum Genet 1986;31:345–352.

37 Komatsu N, Kido A, Oya M: C7 polymorphism in Japanese: New allele C7*8. Hum Hered 1989;39:49–51.

38 Zhang L, Würzner R, Stradmann-Bellinghausen B, Rittner C, Schneider PM: A combined study of human complement C7 IEF and C7 M/N polymorphisms in the Chinese Han population. Exp Clin Immunogenet 1994;11:17–22.

39 Würzner R, Joysey VC, Lachmann PJ: Complement component C7: Assessment of in vivo synthesis after liver transplantation reveals that hepatocytes do not synthesize the majority of human C7. J Immunol 1994;152:4624–4629.

40 Naughton MA, Walport MJ, Würzner R, Carter MJ, Alexander GJM, Goldman JM, Botto M: Organ-specific contribution to circulating C7 levels by the bone marrow and liver in humans. Eur J Immunol 1996;26:2108–2112.

41 Hobart MJ, Lachmann PJ, Calne RY: C6: Synthesis by the liver in vivo. J Exp Med 1977;146:629–630.

42 Høgåsen AKM, Würzner R, Abrahamsen TG, Dierich MP: Human polymorphonuclear leukocytes store large amounts of terminal complement components C7 and C6 which may be released on stimulation. J Immunol 1995;154:4734–4740.

43 Hobart MJ: C7 reference typing and nomenclature recommendations. Complement Inflamm 1990;7:240–242.

44 Würzner R: Deficiencies and polymorphisms of human terminal complement components C6 and C7; PhD thesis, University of Cambridge 1993.

45 Sölder BM, de Stefano GF, Dierich MP, Würzner R: The Cayapa Indians of Ecuador: A genetically isolated group with unexpected complement C7 M/N allele frequencies. Eur J Immunogenet 1996;23:199–203.

46 Würzner R, Tokunaga K, Nitze R, Götze O, Lachmann PJ: C7*N is a hypomorphic allele of the C7 M/N protein polymorphism. Exp Clin Immunogenet 1991;8:177–183.

47 Würzner R, Sölder BM, Prodinger WM, Dierich MP: Complement C7 M/N allotyping in assorted infectious diseases. Exp Clin Immunogenet 1995;12:61–65.

48 Glass D, Raum D, Balavitch D, Kagan E, Rabson A, Schur PH, Alper CA: Inherited deficiency of the sixth component of complement: A silent or null gene. J Immunol 1978;120:538–541.

49 Nishimukai H, Kitamura H, Takeuchi Y, Shinomiya T, Tamaki Y: Three Japanese families with members carrying C7 silent allele (C7*Q0). Possibility for an association between C7*Q0 and C6*B. Hum Hered 1988;38:246–250.

50 Würzner R, Rance N, Potter PC, Hendricks ML, Lachmann PJ, Orren A: C7 M/N protein polymorphism typing applied to inherited deficiencies of human complement proteins C6 and C7. Clin Exp Immunol 1992;89:485–489.

51 Lachmann PJ, Hobart MJ, Woo P: Combined genetic deficiency of C6 and C7 in man. Clin Exp Immunol 1978;33:193–203.

52 Orren A, Würzner R, Potter PC, Fernie BA, Coetzee S, Morgan BP, Lachmann PJ: Properties of a low molecular weight complement component C6 found in human subjects with subtotal C6 deficiency. Immunology 1992;75:10–16.

53 Platonov AE, Würzner R, Beloborodov VB, Jones AM, Troshansky DV, Vershinina IV, Lachmann PJ, Orren A: Paradoxical reconstitution of complement activity following plasma transfusion of an individual with deficiency of the seventh component of complement. Immunology 1994;81:142–148.

54 Würzner R, Platonov AE, Beloborodov VB, Pereverzev AI, Vershinina IV, Fernie BA, Hobart MJ, Lachmann PJ, Orren A: How partial C7 deficiency with chronic and recurrent bacterial infections can mimic total C7 deficiency: Temporary restoration of host C7 level following plasma transfusion. Immunology 1996;88:407–411.

55 Fernie BA, Delbridge G, Hobart MJ: Correlation of a Glu/Ala substitution at position 98 with the complement C6 A/B phenotypes. Hum Mol Genet 1993;2:591–592.

56 Dewald G, Nöthen MM, Cichon S: Polymorphism of human complement component C6: Amino acid substitution (Glu/Ala) within the second thrombospondin repeat differentiates between the two common allotypes C6 A and C6 B. Biochem Biophys Res Commun 1993;194:458–464.

57 Coto E, Dominguez O, Martinez-Naves E, Setien F, Gutierrez V, Lopez-Larrea C: Msp1 polymorphism at the human complement component C6 gene (C6). Nucleic Acids Res 1991;19:194.

58 Potter PC, Warburton C, Würzner R, Orren A, DiScipio R: Association of a 12.5-kilobase allele of the MspI restriction fragment length polymorphism of the C6 gene in patients with total deficiency of the sixth component of complement. Exp Clin Immunogenet 1993;10:38–44.

59 Fernie BA, Finlay A, Price D, Chan E, Orren A, Joysey V, Joysey K, Hobart MJ: Complement C6 and C7 DNA polymorphisms analysed by PCR in seven ethnic groups and characterisation of the C6 Msp I RFLP. Exp Clin Immunogenet 1996;13:92–103.

60 Delbridge GJ: Molecular analysis of the complement component C6 gene; PhD thesis, The Australian National University, Canberra, ACT, 1994.
61 Fernie BA, Hobart MJ: An unususal combined insertion/deletion polymorphism in intron 10 of the complement C6 gene. Hum Genet 1997; 100:104–108.
62 Fernie BA, Würzner R, Unsworth DJ, Tuxworth RI, Hobart MJ: DNA polymorphisms of the complement C6 and C7 genes. Ann Hum Genet 1995;59:163–181.
63 Fernie BA, Hobart MJ: C7 deficiency: Seven further molecular defects and their associated marker haplotypes, including five new polymorphisms. VIIth Complement Genetics Workshop and Conference, Mainz, 21–23 May 1998, Abstract book, P9M.
64 Fernie BA, Würzner R, Orren A, Hobart M: A new intronic polymorphism in the C7 gene 36 bp from the common expressed C7 M/N polymorphism. Ann Hum Genet 1996; 60:179–182.
65 Nishizaka H, Horiuchi T, Zhu Z-B, Fukumori Y, Volanakis JE: Genetic bases of human complement C7 deficiency. J Immunol 1996;157: 4239–4243.
66 DiScipio RG, Chakravarti DN, Müller-Eberhard HJ, Fey GH: The structure of human complement component C7 and the C5b-7 complex. J Biol Chem 1988;263:549–560.
67 Dewald G, Nöthen MM, Rüther K: A common Ser/Thr polymorphism in the perforin-homologous region of complement component C7. Hum Hered 1994;44:301–304.
68 Antonarakis SE and the Nomenclature Working Group: Recommendations for a nomenclature system for human gene mutations. Hum Mutat 1998;11;1–3.
69 Würzner R, Orren A, Lachmann PJ: Inherited deficiencies of the terminal components of human complement. Immunodefic Rev 1992;3: 123–147.
70 Nishizaka H, Horiuchi T, Zhu ZB, Fukumori Y, Nagasawa K, Hayashi K, Krumdieck R, Cobbs CG, Higuchi M, Yasunaga S, Niho Y, Volanakis JE: Molecular bases for inherited human complement component C6 deficiency in two unrelated individuals. J Immunol 1996;156:2309–2315.
71 Hobart MJ, Fernie BA, Fijen CAP, Orren A: The molecular bases of C6 deficiency in the Western Cape, South Africa. VIIth Complement Genetics Workshop and Conference, Mainz, 21–23 May 1998, Abstract book, P10M.
72 Hobart MJ, Fernie BA, Fijen KAPMJ, Orren A: The molecular bases of C6 deficiency in the Western Cape, South Africa. Hum Genet 1998;103:506–512.
73 Zhu ZB, Totemchokchyakarn K, Atkinson TP, Volanakis JE: Molecular defects leading to human complement component C6 deficiency in an African-American family. Clin Exp Immunol 1998;111:91–96.
74 Würzner R, Hobart MJ, Fernie BA, Mewar D, Potter P, Orren A, Lachmann PJ: Molecular basis of subtotal complement C6 deficiency: A carboxyterminally truncated but functionally active C6. J Clin Invest 1995;95:1877–1883.
75 Fernie BA, Würzner R, Orren A, Morgan BP, Potter PC, Platonov AE, Vershinina IV, Shipulin GA, Lachmann PJ, Hobart MJ: Molecular bases of combined subtotal deficiencies of C6 and C7; and their effects in combination with other C6 and C7 deficiencies. J Immunol 1996;157:3648–3657.
76 Fernie BA, Orren A, Sheehan G, Schlesinger M, Hobart MJ: Molecular bases of C7 deficiency: Three different defects. J Immunol 1997;159: 1019–1026.
77 Fernie BA, Hobart MJ: Complement C7 deficiency: Seven further molecular defects and their associated marker haplotypes. Hum Genet 1998;103:513–519.
78 O'Hara AM, Fernie BA, Moran AP, Williams YE, Connaughton JJ, Orren A, Hobart MJ: C7 deficiency in an Irish family; a deletion defect which is predominant in the Irish. Clin Exp Immunol 1998;114:355–361.
79 O'Hara AM, Fernie BA, Orren A, Moran AP, McCluskey DR, Hobart MJ: C7 deficiency in Ireland. Another family with the deletion of C7 exons 7 and 8 and yet another different, undetermined C7 deficiency. Meeting Irish Society Immunology 1997, Galway, 4–5 Sept, 1997.
80 Fijen CA, Kuijper EJ, Hannema AJ, Sjöholm AG, van Putten JP: Complement deficiencies in patients over ten years old with meningococcal disease due to uncommon serogroups. Lancet 1989;ii:585–588.
81 Coto E, Dominguez O, Martinez-Naves E, Urra JM, Gutiérrez V, López-Larrea C: TaqI polymorphism at the human complement component C9 gene. Nucleic Acids Res 1990;18:5581.
82 Rogne S, Mevåg B, Gedde-Dahl T, Myklebost O: Multiple RFLPs of human complement component nine (C9) detected by Taq I. Nucleic Acids Res 1990;18:3112.
83 Witzel-Schlömp K, Rittner C, Schneider PM: DNA polymorphisms in the human complement C9 gene. VIIth Complement Genetics Workshop and Conference, Mainz, 21–23 May 1998, Abstract book, P5M.
84 Weg-Remers S, Brenden M, Schwarz E, Witzel K, Schneider PM, Guerra LK, Rehfeldt IR, Lima MT, Hartmann D, Petzl-Erler ML, deMessias IJT, Mauff G: Major histocompatibility complex (MHC) class III genetics in two Amerindian tribes from Southern Brazil: The Kaingang and the Guarani. Hum Genet 1997;100:548–556.
85 Figueroa JE, Densen P: Infectious diseases associated with complement deficiencies. Clin Microbiol Rev 1991;4:359–395.
86 Fukumori Y, Yoshimura K, Ohnoki S, Yamaguchi H, Akagaki Y, Inai S: A high incidence of C9 deficiency among healthy blood donors in Osaka, Japan. Int Immunol 1989;1:85–89.
87 Hayama K, Sugai N, Tanaka S, Lee S, Kikuchi H, Ito J, Suzuki J, Nagata Y, Kondo H, Harayama O, Tuzuki K, Yoshida S, Fujita M, Ohmori F, Kawai T, Akagaki Y, Inai S: High incidence of C9 deficiency throughout Japan: There are no significant differences in incidence among eight areas of Japan. Int Arch Allergy Appl Immunol 1989;90:400–404.
88 Nagata M, Hara T, Aoki T, Mizuno Y, Akeda H, Inaba S, Tsumoto K, Ueda K: Inherited deficiency of ninth component of complement: An increased risk of meningococcal meningitis. J Pediatr 1989;114:260–264.

89 Fukumori Y, Horiuchi T: Terminal complement component deficiencies in Japan. Exp Clin Immunogenet 1998;15:244–248.
90 Zoppi M, Weiss M, Nydegger UE, Hess T, Späth PJ: Recurrent meningitis in a patient with congenital deficiency of the C9 component of complement. First case of C9 deficiency in Europe. Arch Intern Med 1990;150:2395–2399.
91 Hobart MJ, Fernie BA, Würzner R, Oldroyd RG, Joysey V, Lachmann PJ: Difficulties in the ascertainment of C9 deficiency: Lessons to be drawn from a compound heterozygote C9-deficient subject. Clin Exp Immunol 1997;108:500–506.
92 Witzel-Schlömp K, Hobart MJ, Fernie BA, Orren A, Würzner R, Rittner C, Kaufmann T, Schneider PM: Heterogeneity in the genetic bases of human complement C9 deficiency. Immunogenetics 1998;48:144–147.
93 Horiuchi T, Nishizaka H, Kojima T, Sawabe T, Niho Y, Schneider PM, Inaba S, Sakai K, Hayashi K, Hashimura C, Fukumori Y: A non-sense mutation at Arg95 is predominant in complement 9 deficiency in Japanese. J Immunol 1998;160:1509–1513.
94 Kira R, Ihara K, Takeda H, Gondo K, Hara T: Nonsense mutation in exon 4 of human complement C9 gene is the major cause of Japanese complement C9 deficiency. Hum Genet 1998;102:605–610.
95 Würzner R, Schulze M, Happe L, Franzke A, Bieber FA, Oppermann M, Götze O: Inhibition of terminal complement complex formation and cell lysis by monoclonal antibodies. Complement Inflamm 1991;8:328–340.
96 Würzner R, Orren A, Potter P, Morgan BP, Ponard D, Späth P, Brai M, Schulze M, Happe L, Götze O: Functionally active complement proteins C6 and C7 detected in C6- and C7-deficient individuals. Clin Exp Immunol 1991;83:430–437.
97 Harrison RA, Lachmann PJ: Complement technology; in Weir DM (ed): Handbook of Experimental Immunology, ed 4. Oxford, Blackwell Scientific, 1986 pp. 39.1–39.13.
98 Lengweiler S, Schaller J, Rickli EE: Identification of disulfide bonds in the ninth component (C9) of human complement. FEBS Lett 1996;380:8–12.

Experimental and Clinical Immunogenetics

Exp Clin Immunogenet 1998;15:286–290

Received: September 28, 1998
Accepted: September 30, 1998

G. Geserick
H. Schröder
A. Correns

Institute of Legal Medicine, Humboldt University, Berlin, Germany

Reference Typing Report for Complement Component C6: Protein Typing

Key Words
Complement
C6
Genetic polymorphism
Allotype
C6 nomenclature
Isoelectric focusing
Immunofixation

Abstract
Within the C6/C7/C9 Session of the VIIth Complement Genetics Workshop and Conference, various C6 protein allotypes collected from four laboratories were examined using polyacrylamide gel isoelectric focusing (PAGIF) followed by direct immunofixation. Nineteen different variants including 17 recognized allotypes and introducing two new allotypes were distinguished besides the two common allotypes C6 A and C6 B. They were designated basically according to the previous statement on C6 nomenclature. Details on C6 DNA markers and associations of C6 markers with deficiencies of terminal complement components are published in the preceding paper of this issue.

Introduction

Genetically determined polymorphism of human complement protein C6 was first described in 1975 by Hobart et al. [1]. In 1980, the first statement on the nomenclature of C6 polymorphism was published [2]. Since then, a number of variants have been reported in many human populations. The last reference typing in 1990 established the comparison and designation of these various allotypes [3]. Here we report on a new method to compare various C6 allotypes using polyacrylamide gel isoelectric focusing (PAGIF) followed by direct immunofixation. A total of 19 different allotypes were identified besides 2 common types, including 17 recognized allotypes and introducing 2 new allotypes.

Materials and Methods

Native samples (n = 193) collected from 4 laboratories (Geserick, Berlin; Mauff, Hamburg; Scacchi, Rome; Tokunaga, Tokyo) were subjected to conven-

KARGER
Fax + 41 61 306 12 34
E-Mail karger@karger.ch
www.karger.com

0254–9670/98/0154–0286$17.50/0

Accessible online at:
http://BioMedNet.com/karger

Prof. Dr. med. Gunther Geserick
Institute of Legal Medicine, Medical Faculty (Charité)
Humboldt University, Hannoversche Strasse 6
D–10115 Berlin (Germany)
Tel. +49 30 2093 7311, Fax +49 30 2093 7546

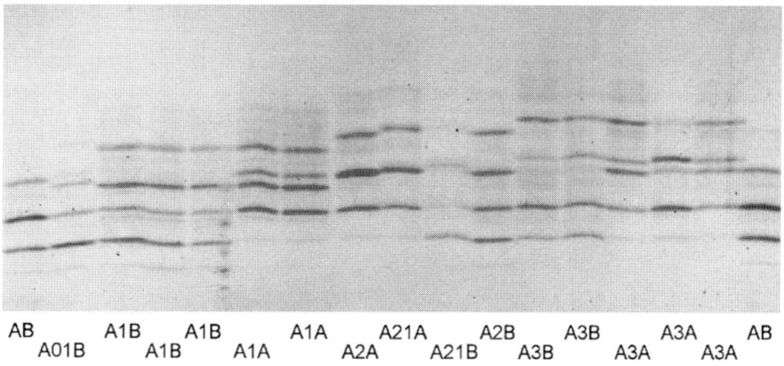

Fig. 1. C6 acidic variants (A) detected by isoelectric focusing and immunofixation. Anode at the top.

Table 1. Method of C6 typing

Samples
Serum samples collected from four laboratories in Berlin (Geserick), Cologne / Hamburg (Mauff), Rome (Scacchi), and Tokyo (Tokunaga)
Isoelectric focusing
Equipment: LKB Multiphor II
Focusing gel: polyacrylamide (T = 5%, C = 3%), 8.2% ampholytes pH 5–6 (LKB / Pharmacia), 0.2 *M* taurine, 2.0 *M* urea, polymerized with TEMED and ammonium persulfate
Separation
– 3-µl sample with filter paper pieces in pH area 7
– Focusing distance of 12.5 cm: 1,600 V, 10 W, 10 mA for a total of 5 h including 1 h prefocusing
Detection
Direct immunofixation
– 0.7 ml antiserum (undiluted) Anti-C6 (Cappel, USA) distributed on the surface of the gel
– Incubation at room temperature for 60 min in a moist chamber
– Washing in 0.9% NaCl solution overnight
– Staining with Serva blue

tional PAGIF followed by direct immunofixation with monospecific antiserum changing the previous techniques of hemolytic overlay [1, 2] or immunoblotting [3, 4]. The details of the typing method are shown in table 1.

Similar or identical variants were compared by running on the same gel, side by side.

Results and Discussion

Figures 1–4 show the patterns of various phenotypes observed in the present reference typing. The C6 patterns obtained with native samples were similar but not identical with those described previously [3, 4]. In homozygous phenotypes, two major bands and at least one acidic and one basic minor band

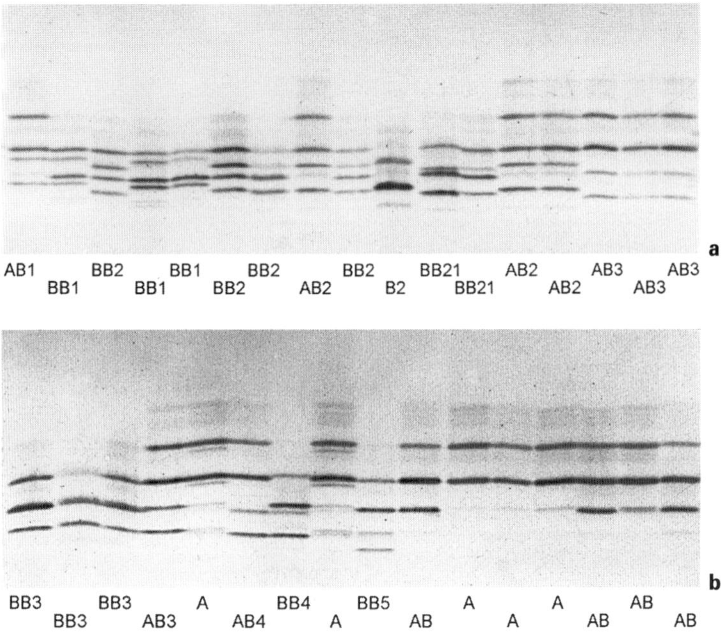

Fig. 2. a C6 basic variants (B1, B2, B21, B3) detected by isoelectric focusing and immunofixation. Anode at the top. **b** C6 basic variants (B3, B4, B5) detected by isoelectric focusing and immunofixation. Anode at the top.

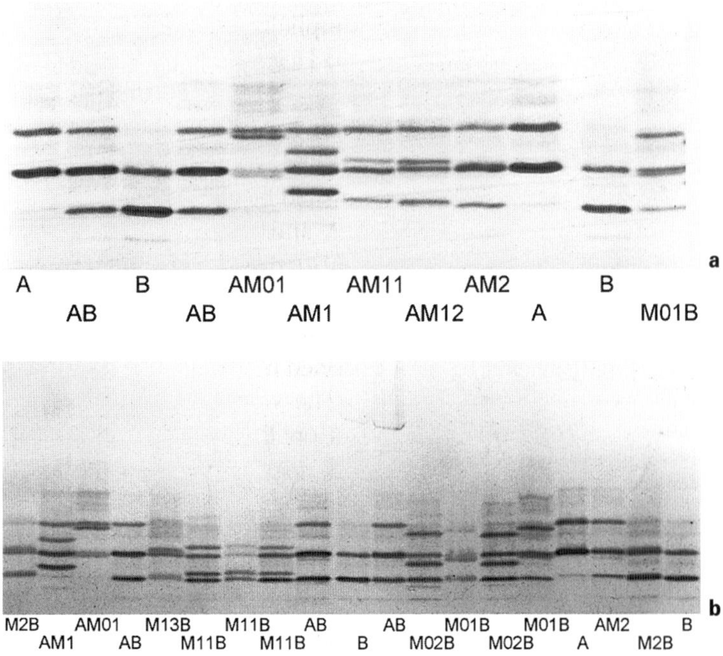

Fig. 3. a C6 intermediate variants (M) including the new allotype M12 detected by isoelectric focusing and immunofixation. Anode at the top. **b** C6 intermediate variants (M) including the new allotype M13 detected by isoelectric focusing and immunofixation. Anode at the top.

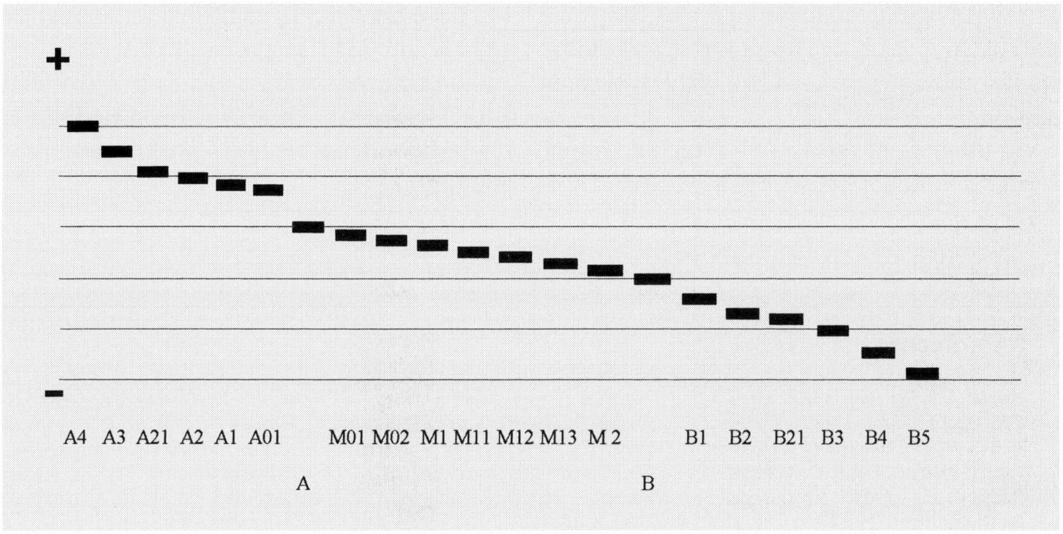

Fig. 4. Schematic representation of presently identified C6 variants (only the major bands are shown). Anode at the top.

were observed. A combination of three or four major bands and additional minor bands was observed in heterozygous phenotypes. In most cases, the untreated samples could be typed easily because of the simplicity and clarity of the patterns, this included aged samples as well.

The results of the reference typing are summarized in table 2 and figure 4. In total, 19 different allotypes were distinguished besides the two common allotypes C6 A and C6 B. Seventeen variants of them identified in the previous paper on C6 reference typing [3] are included in the present study. For many variants, inheritance has been established in family studies [reviewed in ref. 3]. The variants were designated generally based on the nomenclature statement in 1980 [2], respectively 1990 [3], except for 2 samples. We have relabeled these 2 intermediate allotypes between C6 A and C6 M1, named C6 M91 and C6 M92 [5, 6], M01 (previously M92) and M02 (previously M91), to put these variants

Table 2. C6 variants identified in the main C6 reference laboratory (Berlin)

Allotype	Samples
A4	1
A3	5
A21	2
A2	15
A1	37
A01	1
M01 (previous M92)	3
M02 (previous M91)	2
M1	3
M11	5
M12 (new)	1
M13 (new)	2
M2	41
B1	18
B2	36
B21	3
B3	15
B4	2
B5	1
Total	193

in the same alphanumeric order as the variants of C6 A or C6 B. This proposal was unanimously accepted in the C6/C7/C9 workshop session.

In the present reference typing, two intermediate variants between C6 M11 and C6 M2 have been newly identified and designated M12 and M13, respectively (fig. 3a, b).

Until further notice, the main C6 Reference Typing Laboratory will be in Berlin, but reference samples are also stored in Innsbruck and Mainz [7].

References

1 Hobart MJ, Lachmann PJ, Alper CA: Polymorphism of human C6; in Peeters H (ed): Protides of the Biological Fluids. 22nd Colloqium, Brugge 1974. Oxford, Pergamon Press, 1975, pp 575–580.

2 Mauff G, Alper CA, Hobart M, Kühnl P, Kunstmann G, Meo T, Olving JH, Rittner C: Statement on the nomenclature of human C6 polymorphism. Immunobiology 1980;158:139–143.

3 Tokunaga K, Jin F, Mauff G, Nishimukai H, Simeoni E, Suzuki K, Weber W: C6 reference typing report. Complement Inflamm 1990;7:234–239.

4 Tokunaga K, Yukiyama Y, Omoto K: Polymorphism of the complement C6 in Japanese. J Immunogenet 1983;10:419–424.

5 Tokunaga K, Yamamura N, Omoto K: An immunoblotting technique for complement C6 typing: Three new variants. Jpn J Hum Genet 1984;29:415–419.

6 Washio K, Tokunaga K, Omoto K, Misawa S: Human C7 polymorphism: Classification and association analysis with C6. Jpn J Hum Genet 1986;31:345–352.

7 Würzner R, Witzel-Schlömp K, Tokunaga K, Fernie BA, Hobart MJ, Orren A: Reference typing report for complement components C6, C7 and C9 including mutations leading to deficiencies. Exp Clin Immunogenet 1998;15:268–285.

Experimental and Clinical Immunogenetics

Exp Clin Immunogenet 1998;15:291–294

Received: September 4, 1998
Accepted: September 14, 1998

Reference Typing Report for Complement Receptor 1 (CR1)

J.M. Moulds[a], *M. Brai*[b]
J. Cohen[c], *A. Cortelazzo*[d]
M. Cuccia[d], *M. Lin*[e]
S. Sadallah[f], *J. Schifferli*[f]
V. Bala Subramanian[i]
L. Truedsson[g], *G.W. Wu*[h]
F. Zhang[i], *J.P. Atkinson*[i]

[a] University of Texas-Houston Medical School, Houston, Tex., USA;
[b] Università degli Studi di Palermo, Italy;
[c] Centre Hospitalier Universitaire de Reims, France;
[d] Università di Pavia, Italy;
[e] Mackay Hospital, Taipei, Taiwan;
[f] University of Basel, Switzerland;
[g] Lund University Hospital, Lund, Sweden;
[h] Shen-Zhen Blood Center, Shen-Zhen, PRC;
[i] Washington University Medical School, St. Louis, Mo., USA

Key Words
Complement receptor
CR1
CD35
Polymorphism

Abstract

A total of 100 Chinese blood donors (50 from Shen-Zhen and 50 from Taiwan) were studied by the participants in addition to 9 reference samples. A new nomenclature for the CR1 structural alleles was recommended by the participants which would use a numbering system, e.g. CR1*1. The structural allele frequencies in the Chinese were: CR1*1 (190 kD) 0.96, CR1*2 (220 kD) 0.03, CR1*3 (160 kD) 0.01 and CR1*4 (250 kD) 0.00. The *Hin*dIII expression polymorphism was also studied and the high expressing allele had a gene frequency of 0.71 while the low expressor gene frequency was 0.28. Erythrocyte copy numbers were quantified and compared between laboratories with good correlation (R = 0.55–0.88). The mean (± SD) erythrocyte copy number was 463 (± 229) in the Taiwan donors and 446 (± 207) in the Mainland Chinese.

Introduction

During the organization of the section for the investigation of complement receptor type 1 (CR1) several aims were outlined. The consensus was that gene frequencies should be established in populations that have yet to be studied. Accordingly, it was decided that a group of 100 Chinese donors would be tested for the structural alleles and the high (*H*) and low (*L*) expression alleles. Also, the red cells would be tested for actual CR1 copy numbers (E CR1). Subsequently 50 healthy blood donors were obtained through Dr. Marie Lin in Taiwan and 50 from Dr. Wu in the People's Republic of China. Both genomic DNA and

KARGER

Fax + 41 61 306 12 34
E-Mail karger@karger.ch
www.karger.com

0254–9670/98/0154–0291$17.50/0

Accessible online at:
http://BioMedNet.com/karger

Dr. Joann M. Moulds
University of Texas
Houston Medical School, 6431 Fannin
Houston, TX 77030 (USA)
Tel. +1 713 500 6889, Fax +1 713 500 0580

Table 1. Summary of the CR1 structural alleles and expression polymorphisms for the standard donor samples

Donor No.	Race	CR1 size	*Hin*dIII RFLP
980145	Caucasian	190,220	HH
980146	Caucasian	190,190	HL
980147	Caucasian	190,220	HH
980148	Caucasian	160,190	HL
980149	Caucasian	190,190	LL
980150	Caucasian	190,220	HH
980151	African-American	190,250	HH
980154	African-American	160,190	HH
980156	African-American	220,220	HH

The CR1 molecular weights are given in kilodaltons on non-reduced gels. Approximately 30 kD should be added to the above results if run under reducing conditions.

red blood cells were sent to the participants. It was also felt that a group of known 'standard' donor samples be sent to each participating lab in order to compare results and establish nomenclature. These samples were supplied by the coordinators (J.M.M. and J.P.A.).

Standard Donors

A total of 9 'standard' samples were obtained, 8 were from healthy controls and 1 from a patient diagnosed with systemic lupus erythematosus. Six of the donors were Caucasian and 3 were African-American. The donors represented all 4 of the published CR1 structural alleles. In addition they represented all three expression genotypes, i.e. homozygous *HH* or *LL* and heterozygous (*HL*). The results are summarized in table 1.

The Knops blood group antigens are expressed on CR1 [1]. These include the 'high-frequency' alleles: Kn^a, McC^a, Sl^a and Yk^a. Donor 980145 was chosen because the 220-kD protein does not express the McC^a blood group antigen. All other donors are positive for the Knops blood group antigens.

Donor 980148 was chosen because the 190-kD allele is only weakly expressed and is inherited with the *L* allele as shown by a family study. All participants doing structural allele testing reported similar results. Donor 980149 also has weak expression of the 190 kD protein but is homozygous *LL*. In addition, this donor is the original Knops null phenotype known as the 'Helgeson' type [2].

Other donors representing the 160-, 220- and 250-kD phenotypes were included and the workshop participants (fig. 1) detected all of them. On occasion, cleavage fragments of CR1 were observed (lanes 3, 4, 5, 7, 8, 9) by those participants using Western blotting technique that were not seen using immunoprecipitation. Some monoclonal antibodies, e.g. E11, J3D3 more readily detected these bands while others (J3B11) did not.

In reporting the results, the participants referred to each of these alleles using the current A, B, C, D terminology. However, it was agreed that this was, at times, confusing since the long homologous repeats (LHR) of CR1 have also been referred to as A, B, C, D. A proposal was made to make the nomenclature more similar to other complement compo-

Table 2. Proposed terminology for CR1 alleles

New name	Old name	CR1 size, kD[a]	Old name	CR1 size, kD[b]
CR1*1	CR1-A	190	F	220
CR1*2	CR1-B	220	S	250
CR1*3	CR1-C	160	F'	190
CR1*4	CR1-D	250	None	280

a Under non-reducing conditions.
b Under reducing conditions.

nent nomenclatures, e.g. C4. This would also allow for expansion pending the molecular identification of the blood group alleles. Therefore, the CR1 participants unanimously recommend that the alleles be named in order of decreasing gene frequency (based on several studies of different ethnic groups). The new and old terminology are shown in table 2.

Chinese Donors

There was very good agreement between the laboratories that studied the CR1 size variants of the Chinese samples. Only 4 discrepancies (total n = 100) were noted; 3 of them were due to the failure to detect a 220-kD protein that was weakly expressed. CR1*1 was the most frequent allele (0.96) while the others were uncommon (CR1*2 = 0.03) or rare (CR1*3 = 0.01 and CR1*4 = 0). The CR1*2 allele was distributed equally between the Taiwan and the Mainland China donors while the 2 examples of CR1*3 were found in the Taiwan samples.

The high/low alleles were studied both by Southern blot and by a PCR-RFLP method with excellent agreement between them. Eight of 54 samples or 15% were homozygous for *LL* which is higher than reported in other populations. The gene frequencies were *H* = 0.71 and *L* = 0.28. When comparing E CR1 copy number to the *H/L* polymorphism, the *HH* individuals had a higher mean number than the *LL*; however, there was considerable overlap in the *HL* group. The assays used to determine copy number are described below. Suggested methods for the CR1 size determination [3] and the *Hin*dIII RFLP [4] are given under References.

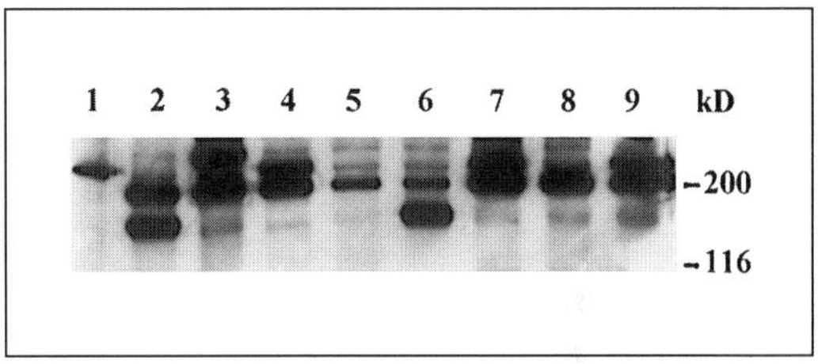

Fig. 1. Chemiluminescence Western blot using monoclonal anti-CR1 (J3D3) and the procedure outlined in reference 3 (pg 79–80) to determine CR1 size polymorphism. Lane 1 = 980156; lane 2 = 980154; lane 3 = 980151; lane 4 = 980150; lane 5 = 980149; lane 6 = 980148; lane 7 = 980147; lane 8 = 980146; lane 9 = 980145.

CR1 Copy Number

All 9 standard samples and the 100 test samples (50 each from Taiwan and Mainland China) described above were analyzed for erythrocyte CR1 copy number. Four different laboratories analyzed the 'standards' and the test samples from Taiwan. The test samples from Mainland China wcrc tcstcd by onc laboratory (JPA). Three of the laboratories used ELISA-based techniques whereas the 4th one used flow cytometry. For ELISA, the antibodies (capture/detection) used were: 3D9/E11-HRP (JPA), E11/J3B11 (JC) and 3D9/J3D3 (JS). mAb To5 was used for FACS analysis (LT).

There was an expected correlation between the four laboratories and the two techniques for erythrocyte CR1 copy numbers on the 'standards'. There was also agreement between the laboratories on the CR1 copy numbers for the test erythrocytes from China (r = 0.55–0.88). Overall E CR1 in the Chinese samples were normally distributed with a range of 27–1,039 and a mean ± SD of 463 ± 229 (Taiwan) and 446 ± 207 (Mainland China). Two samples (980197, 980208), both from Mainland China, were notable for copy numbers of 28 and 27 E CR1, lower than our 'Helgeson' phenotype standard.

The consensus view on erythrocyte CR1 copy number was: (a) FACS analysis, compared to ELISA-based methods, is equally sensitive and acceptable for determining relative copy numbers of CR1 on erythrocytes. (b) E CR1 copy numbers, in the two Chinese populations, were within the published range and the means were similar to those of other ethnic groups. (c) Further study of the 2 individuals with very low E CR1 copies will be of interest. (d) Because of the internal homology within CR1, the number of epitopes for many of the detection antibodies will vary among the polymorphic forms of CR1 [5]. The potential, therefore, for underestimation of copy numbers for the CR1*3 form or overestimation for CR1*2 and CR1*4 should be borne in mind.

References

1 Moulds JM, Nickells MW, Moulds JJ, Brown MC, Atkinson JP: The C3b/C4b receptor is recognized by the Knops, McCoy, Swain-Langley, and York blood group antisera. J Exp Med 1991;173:1159–1163.

2 Moulds JM, Moulds JJ, Brown M, Atkinson JP: Antiglobulin testing for CR1-related (Knops/McCoy/Swain-Langley/York) blood group antigens: Negative and weak reactions are caused by variable expression of CR1. Vox Sang 1991;62: 230–235.

3 Nickells MW, Atkinson JP: Identification, functional assessment, and quantitation of receptors and membrane regulatory proteins whose ligands are C3 and C4; in Dodds AW, Sim RB (eds): Complement: A Practical Approach. Oxford, IRL Press at Oxford University Press, 1997, pp 68–91.

4 Cornillet P, Philbert F, Kazatchkine MD, Cohen JHM: Genomic determination of the CR1 (CD35) density polymorphism on erythrocytes using polymerase chain reaction amplification and *Hin*dIII restriction enzyme digestion. J Immunol Methods 1991;136:193–197.

5 Nickells M, Hauhart R, Krych M, Bala Subramanian V, Geoghegan-Barek K, Marsh H, Atkinson JP: Mapping of epitopes for 20 monoclonal antibodies to CR1. Clin Exp Immunol 1998;112:27–33.

Experimental and Clinical
Immunogenetics

Exp Clin Immunogenet 1998;15:295

Rother K, Till GO, Hänsch GM (eds)

The Complement System

Springer, Berlin 1998
XX + 564 pp.; DEM 248.–
ISBN 3–540–61894–5

Complement provides an important host defence system involved in a multitude of immune reactions, including opsonisation of micro-organisms, enhancement of the inflammatory response, clearance of immune complexes and cell lysis. The first English edition of *The Complement System*, following an earlier German one, was published in 1987 and was well received by biochemists and immunologists working in the complement field. Through the years, it became a standard text book in many laboratories. After 11 years, it was time to publish the second edition, considering the multiple new developments in this area.

This second edition not only represents a thorough revision of the 1987 edition, but also focusses much more on biological functions (chapter 2, including the topics 'Host defence', 'Reproduction' and 'Network Interactions') and the role of complement in pathological conditions (chapter 3, including the topics 'Deficiencies', 'Transplantation' and 'Biocompatibility').

The editors and authors, all outstanding scientists in the complement field, have succeeded in providing a broad and comprehensive textbook which can be recommended to basic researchers and scientists working in medical microbiology or immunology. For clinicians, I especially recommend chapter 5 on 'The Clinical Laboratory: Testing the Complement System', which details virtually all available complement assays. However, this very impressive chapter alone does not compensate for the overall lack of clinical orientation. Although clinical subjects are addressed, they are scattered from a clinical point of view, e.g. sections 2.2, 3.3 and 3.4, which are important for nephrologists. Very short structural sections on 'Complement in Dermatological Diseases' or 'Complement in Renal Diseases' could have told the clinician which chapters are important for him/her and how they are interconnected with each other without necessarily going into detail in that section.

This comprehensive book has also incorporated the newly discovered 'MBLectin Pathway', not only by introducing this system in one excellently written section, but also by referring to it throughout the book in different sections: I was also delighted to see a chapter on 'Complement Manipulation in vivo' (chapter 4). However, this chapter, although very nicely written, is a bit short considering the many new developments in this field, e.g. complement inhibitory antibodies and the preliminary use of complement regulators in xenotransplantation, which could have been mentioned there as well.

Unfortunately, the previous chapter on 'Complement Genetics' was completely omitted from the second edition, without even referring to this topic. Textbooks do get thicker with each edition, so some topics have to be omitted, but I would not have left out this chapter completely (not only my very personal opinion!).

Many citations help the interested reader to gain more information on the various subjects and most chapters, but not all, are well illustrated.

In conclusion, this is an excellent text book for the experienced clinician or researcher as well as for the young scientist working with or only interested in complement.

Reinhard Würzner, Innsbruck

KARGER
Fax + 41 61 306 12 34
E-Mail karger@karger.ch
www.karger.com

0254–9670/98/0154–0295$17.50/0

Accessible online at:
http://BioMedNet.com/karger

Author Index Vol. 15, No. 4, 1998

Experimental and Clinical Immunogenetics

(B) = Book Review

Subject Index Vol. 15, No. 4, 1998

KARGER

Fax + 41 61 306 12 34
E-Mail karger@karger.ch
www.karger.com

Accessible online at:
http://BioMedNet.com/karger

Author Index Vol. 15, 1998

Experimental and Clinical Immunogenetics

(B) = Book Review

KARGER
Fax +41 61 306 12 34
E-Mail karger@karger.ch
www.karger.com

Accessible online at:
http://BioMedNet.com/karger

Subject Index Vol. 15, 1998

Experimental and Clinical Immunogenetics

KARGER

Fax + 41 61 306 12 34
E-Mail karger@karger.ch
www.karger.com
Accessible online at:
http://BioMedNet.com/karger

Vol. 15, 1998

Experimental and Clinical Immunogenetics

KARGER

Basel · Freiburg · Paris · London · New York · New Delhi · Bangkok · Singapore · Tokyo · Sydney

KARGER

S. Karger
Medical and Scientific Publishers
Basel · Freiburg · Paris · London
New York · New Delhi · Bangkok
Singapore · Tokyo · Sydney

Drug Dosage
The authors and the publisher have exerted every effort to ensure that drug selection and dosage set forth in this text are in accord with current recommendations and practice at the time of publication. However, in view of ongoing research, changes in government regulations, and the constant flow of information relating to drug therapy and drug reactions, the reader is urged to check the package insert for each drug for any change in indications and dosage and for added warnings and precautions. This is particularly important when the recommended agent is a new and/or infrequently employed drug.

Printed in Switzerland on acid-free paper by
Reinhardt Druck, Basel

Contents Vol. 15, 1998

Experimental and Clinical Immunogenetics

No. 1

No. 2

KARGER

Fax + 41 61 306 12 34
E-Mail karger@karger.ch
www.karger.com

Access to full text and tables of contents, including tentative ones for forthcoming issues:
www.karger.com/journals/eci/eci_bk.htm